TESTING TREATMENTS
BETTER RESEARCH FOR BETTER HEALTHCARE

TESTING TREATMENTS
BETTER RESEARCH FOR BETTER HEALTHCARE

Imogen Evans, Hazel Thornton & Iain Chalmers

foreword by Ben Goldacre

We dedicate this book to William Silverman (1917–2004), who encouraged us repeatedly to challenge authority.

Testing Treatments
Better Research for Better Healthcare

First published in 2006 by The British Library
This reprint edition published 2010 by Pinter & Martin Ltd

British Library Cataloguing in Publication Data
A catalogue record for this book is available from the British Library

ISBN 978-1-905177-35-6

Typeset at The Spartan Press Limited, Lymington, Hants
Designed by Andrew Shoolbred
Printed and bound in the EU by Megaprint, Turkey

This book has been printed on paper that is sourced and harvested from sustainable forests and is FSC accredited

Pinter & Martin Ltd
6 Effra Parade
London SW2 1PS
Telephone 020-7737 6868
info@pinterandmartin.com
www.pinterandmartin.com

CONTENTS

ABOUT THE AUTHORS

Imogen Evans practised and lectured in medicine in Canada and the UK before turning to medical journalism at *The Lancet*. From 1996 to 2005 she worked for the Medical Research Council, latterly in research ethics, and has represented the UK government on the Council of Europe Biomedical Ethics Committee.

Hazel Thornton, after undergoing routine mammography, was invited to join a clinical trial, but the inadequate patient information led to her refusal. However, it also encouraged her advocacy for public involvement in research to achieve outcomes relevant to patients. She has written and spoken extensively on this topic.

Iain Chalmers practised medicine in the UK and Palestine before becoming a health services researcher and directing the National Perinatal Epidemiology Unit and then the UK Cochrane Centre. Since 2003 he has coordinated the James Lind Initiative, promoting better controlled trials for better healthcare, particularly through greater public involvement.

ACKNOWLEDGEMENTS

We thank Tony Warshaw for encouraging us to write *Testing Treatments*. We are indebted to Richard Ashcroft, Patricia Atkinson, Hilda Bastian, Michael Baum, Joan Box, Noreen Caine, Harry Cayton, Jan Chalmers, Alison Chapple, Mike Clarke, John Critchlow, Ben Djulbegovic, George Ebers, Robin Fox, Jo Garcia, Paul Glasziou, Bec Hanley, Elina Hemminki, Andrew Herxheimer, Tony Hope, Les Irwig, Debbie Kennett, Richard Lindley, Margaret McCartney, Wilson Ng, Ann Oakley, Michael Parker, Sophie Petit-Zeman, Uccio Querci della Rovere, Nick Ross, Eileen and David Ruxton, Harvey Schipper, Lara Speicher and Belinda Wilkinson for helpful comments on earlier drafts of our manuscript, and to Theo Chalmers for designing the cover of the book. Iain Chalmers is grateful to the Medical Research Council and the NHS Research and Development Programme for support.

FOREWORD

Medicine shouldn't be about authority, and the most important question anyone can ask on any claim is simple: "how do you know?" This book is about the answer to that question.

There has been a huge shift in the way that people who work in medicine relate to patients. In the distant past, "communications skills training", such as it was, consisted of how *not* to tell your patient they were dying of cancer. Today we teach students – and this is a direct quote from the hand-outs – how to "work collaboratively with the patient towards an optimum health outcome". Today, if they wish, at medicine's best, patients are involved in discussing and choosing their own treatments.

For this to happen, it's vital that everyone understands how we know if a treatment works, how we know if it has harms, and how we weigh benefits against harms to determine the risk. Sadly doctors can fall short on this, as much as anybody else. Even more sadly, there is a vast army out there, queuing up to mislead us.

First and foremost in this gallery of rogues, we can mislead ourselves. Most diseases have a natural history, getting better and worse in cycles, or at random: because of this, anything you do, if you act when symptoms are at their worst, might make a treatment seem to be effective, because you were going to get better anyway.

The placebo effect, similarly, can be a deep source of misleading mischief: people really can get better, in some cases, simply from taking a dummy pill with no active ingredients, and by believing their treatments to be effective. As Robert M Pirsig said, in *Zen and the Art of Motorcycle Maintenance*: "the real purpose of the scientific method is to make sure nature hasn't misled you into thinking you know something you actually don't know".

But then there are the people who brandish scientific studies. If there is one key message from this book – and it is a phrase I have borrowed and used endlessly myself – it is the concept of a "fair test". Not all trials are born the same, because there are so many ways that a piece of scientific research can be biased, and erroneously give what someone, somewhere thinks should be the "right" answer.

Sometimes evidence can be distorted through absent-mindedness, or the purest of motives, for all that motive matters. Doctors, patients, professors, nurses, occupational therapists, and managers can all become wedded to the idea that one true treatment, in which they have invested so much personal energy, is golden.

Sometimes evidence can be distorted for other reasons. It would be wrong to fall into shallow conspiracy theories about the pharmaceutical industry: they have brought huge, lifesaving advances. But there is a lot of money at stake in some research, and for reasons you will see in this book, 90% of trials are conducted by industry. This can be a problem, when studies funded by industry are four times more likely to have a positive result for the sponsor's drug than independently funded trials. It costs up to $800m to bring a new drug to market, and while that money is spent over ten years of development, the drug could fail to shine at any stage in the process. If the stakes are so high, sometimes the ideals of a fair test can fail.[1]

Equally, the way that evidence is communicated can be distorted, and misleading. Sometimes this can be in the presentation of facts and figures, telling only part of the story, glossing over flaws, and "cherry picking" the scientific evidence which shows one treatment in a particular light.

But in popular culture, there can be more interesting processes at play. We have an understandable desire for miracle cures, even though research is frequently about modest improvements, shavings of risk, and close judgement calls. In the media, all too often this can be thrown aside in a barrage of words like "cure", "miracle", "hope", "breakthrough", and "victim".[2]

At a time when so many are so keen to take control of their own lives, and be involved in decisions about their own healthcare, it is sad to see so much distorted information, as it can only disempower. Sometimes these distortions are around a specific drug: the presentation in the UK media of Herceptin as a miracle cure for breast cancer is perhaps the most compelling recent example.[3]

Sometimes, though, in promoting their own treatments, and challenging the evidence against them, zealots and their friends in the media can do even greater damage, by actively undermining the public's very understanding of *how we know* if something is good for us, or bad for us.

Homoeopathy sugar pills perform no better than dummy sugar pills when compared by the most fair tests. But when confronted with this evidence, homoeopaths argue that there is something wrong with the whole notion of doing a trial, that there is some complicated reason why their pills, uniquely among pills, cannot be tested. Politicians, when confronted with evidence that their favoured teaching programme for preventing teenage pregnancy has failed, may fall into the same kind of special pleading. In reality, as this book will show, any claim made about an intervention having an effect can be subjected to a transparent fair test.[4]

Sometimes these distortions can go even deeper into undermining the public's understanding. A recent "systematic review" of all the most fair and unbiased tests showed there was no evidence that taking antioxidant vitamin pills can prolong life (in fact, they may even shorten it). With this kind of summary – as explained beautifully in this book – clear rules are followed, describing where to look for evidence, what evidence can be included, and how its quality should be assessed. But when systematic reviews produce a result that challenges the claims of antioxidant supplement pill companies, newspapers and magazines are filled with false criticisms, arguing that, for reasons of political allegiance or frank corruption, that favourable evidence has been deliberately ignored, and so on.[5]

This is unfortunate. The notion of systematic review – looking at the totality of evidence – is quietly one of the most important innovations in medicine over the past 30 years. In defending their business, but undermining our access to these ideas, these journalists and pill companies do us all a great disservice.

And that is the rub. There are many reasons to read this book. At the simplest level, it will help you make your own decisions about your own health in a much more informed way. If you work in medicine, the chapters that follow will probably stand head and shoulders above any teaching you had in evidence-based medicine. At the population level, if more people understand how to make fair comparisons, and see whether one intervention is better than another, then as the authors argue, instead of sometimes fearing research, the public might actively campaign to be more involved in reducing uncertainties about the treatments that matter to them.

But there is one final reason to read this book, to learn the "tricks of the trade", and that reason has nothing to do with practicality: the plain fact is, this stuff is interesting, and beautiful, and clever. In this book it's explained better than anywhere else I've ever seen, because of the people who wrote it, their knowledge, their experience, and – it would be wrong to say "oddly for a book about methodology", although it's probably true – their empathy.

Read on.

Ben Goldacre
27th January 2010

[1] Joel Lexchin et al., "Pharmaceutical industry sponsorship and research outcome and quality: systematic review," *BMJ* 326, no. 7400 (May 29, 2003): 1167–1170.

[2] Gary Schwitzer et al., "What Are the Roles and Responsibilities of the Media in Disseminating Health Information?," PLoS Med 2, no. 7 (July 26, 2005): e215.

[3] Paul M Wilson et al., "Deconstructing media coverage of trastuzumab (Herceptin): an analysis of national newspaper coverage," *J R Soc Med* 101, no. 3 (March 1, 2008): 125–132.

[4] Shang A et al., "Are the clinical effects of homoeopathy placebo effects? Comparative study of placebo-controlled trials of homoeopathy and allopathy," *Lancet* 366, no. 9487 (September 27, 2005): 726–732.

[5] Bjelakovic G, Nikolova D, Gluud LL, Simonetti RG, Gluud C. Antioxidant supplements for prevention of mortality in healthy participants and patients with various diseases. *Cochrane Database of Systematic Reviews* 2008, Issue 2. Art. No.: CD007176. DOI: 10.1002/14651858.CD007176.

FOREWORD TO THE FIRST PRINTING

This book is good for our health. It shines light on the mysteries of how life and death decisions are made. It shows how those judgements are often badly flawed and it sets a challenge for doctors across the globe to mend their ways.

Yet it accomplishes this without unnecessary scares; and it warmly admires much of what modern medicine has achieved. Its ambitions are always to improve medical practice, not disparage it.

My own first insight into entrenched sloppiness in medicine came in the 1980s when I was invited to be a lay member of a consensus panel set up to judge best practice in the treatment of breast cancer. I was shocked (and you may be too when you read more about this issue in Chapter 2). We took evidence from leading researchers and clinicians and discovered that some of the most eminent consultants worked on hunch or downright prejudice and that a woman's chance of survival, and of being surgically disfigured, greatly depended on who treated her and what those prejudices were. One surgeon favoured heroic mutilation, another preferred simple lump removal, a third opted for aggressive radiotherapy, and so on. It was as though the age of scientific appraisal had passed them by.

Indeed, it often had, and for many doctors it still does. Although things have improved, many gifted, sincere and skilful medical practitioners are surprisingly ignorant about what constitutes good scientific evidence. They do what they do because that is what they were taught in medical school, or because it is what other doctors do, or because in their experience it works. But personal experience, though beguiling, is often terribly misleading – as this book shows, with brutal clarity.

Some doctors say it is naïve to apply scientific rigour to the treatment of individual patients. Medicine, they assert, is both a science and an art. But, noble as that sounds, it is a contradiction in terms. Of course medical knowledge is finite and with any individual the complexities are almost infinite, so there is always an element of uncertainty. In practice, good medicine routinely requires good guesswork. But too often in the past many medical professionals have blurred the distinction between guessing and good evidence. Sometimes they even proclaim certainty when there is really considerable doubt. They eschew reliable data because they are not sure how to assess them.

This book explains the difference between personal experience and more complex, but better ways of distinguishing what works from what does not and what is safe from what is not. Insofar as it can, it avoids technical terms, and promotes plain English expressions like 'fair tests'. It warns that science, like everything else in human affairs, is prone to error and bias (through mistakes, vanity or – especially pernicious in medicine – the demands of commerce); but it reminds us that, even so, it is the meticulous approach of science that has created almost all of the most conspicuous advances in human knowledge. Doctors (and media-types, like me) should stop disparaging clinical research as 'trials on human guinea-pigs'; on the contrary there is a moral imperative for all practitioners to promote fair tests to their patients and for patients to participate.

This is an important book for anyone concerned about their own or their family's health, or the politics of health. Patients are often seen as the recipients of healthcare, rather than participants. The task ahead is as much for us, the lay public in whose name medicine is practised and from whose purse medical practitioners are paid, as for doctors and medical researchers. If we are passive consumers of medicine we will never drive up standards. If we prefer simplistic answers we will get pseudoscience. If we do not promote the rigorous testing of treatments we will get pointless and sometimes dangerous treatment along with the stuff that really works.

This book contains a manifesto for improving things, and patients are at its heart. But it is an important book for doctors, medical students, and researchers too – all would benefit from its lessons. In an ideal world, it would be compulsory reading for every journalist, and available to every patient, because if doctors are inadequate at weighing up scientific evidence, in general we, whose very mortality depends on this, are worse.

One thing I promise: if this subject of testing treatments is new to you, once you have read this book you will never feel quite the same about your doctor's advice again.

Nick Ross
TV and radio presenter and journalist
16 November 2005

INTRODUCTION

There is no way to know when our observations about complex events in nature are complete. Our knowledge is finite, Karl Popper emphasised, but our ignorance is infinite. In medicine, we can never be certain about the consequences of our interventions, we can only narrow the area of uncertainty. This admission is not as pessimistic as it sounds: claims that resist repeated energetic challenges often turn out to be quite reliable. Such "working truths" are the building blocks for the reasonably solid structures that support our everyday actions at the bedside.

William A. Silverman. *Where's the evidence?* 1998[1]

We have been colleagues for many years, sharing not only professional camaraderie but also a deep-seated conviction that medical treatments, whether new or old, should be based on sound evidence. Our collective experience of healthcare and healthcare research suggests this is often not the case. And that is what encouraged us to write this book.

IE's curiosity about the evidence underpinning the treatments she prescribed to patients was heightened during her career in medical research. When she became a medical journalist at *The Lancet* she encountered flagrant attempts by some pharmaceutical companies and researchers to economise with the truth by distorting or embellishing their research results. HT's unexpected invitation to participate in a clinical trial of doubtful quality made her realise that she ought to be an active participant in the quest for progress concerning her treatment, not a more or less passive recipient of care. She went on to campaign vigorously for collaboration between health professionals and patients to ensure worthwhile research with good quality patient information. IC's obsession with rigorous assessment of the effects of the things that doctors do to their patients began when he was working in a Palestinian refugee camp: some of his patients seemed to be dying because he was practising in ways that he had been taught at medical school. Since then he has strenuously promoted the view that decisions in healthcare should be informed by unbiased evidence from relevant research, particularly the results of systematic reviews of controlled trials.

Every year, studies into the effects of treatments generate a mountain of results. Sadly, much of this research fails to address the needs of patients, and even when it does, the evidence is often unreliable. We hope our book will point the way to wider understanding of how treatments can and should be tested fairly. This is not a best treatments guide to the effects of individual therapies. Rather, we highlight issues that are fundamental to ensuring that research is soundly based and designed to answer questions that matter to patients and the health professionals to whom they turn for help.

In Chapter 1 we describe how some new treatments have had harmful effects that were unexpected; the hoped-for effects of others failed to materialise; and some predictions that treatments would not work were proved wrong. Furthermore, some useful results of research have not been applied in practice. In Chapter 2 we highlight the fact that many commonly used treatments and screening tests have not been adequately evaluated. Chapter 3 gives some 'technical details' – here we outline the basis for fair testing of treatments, emphasising the im- portance of paying attention to reducing potential biases and taking account of the play of chance; this chapter also introduces concepts such as randomised clinical trials and placebos, and the need to review systematically all the relevant evidence. In Chapter 4 we describe some of the numerous uncertainties that pervade almost every aspect of healthcare, and how to tackle them. Chapter 5 contrasts the key differences between good, bad, and unnecessary research into the effects of treatments. In Chapter 6 we point out how much of the research that is done is distorted by commercial and academic priorities and fails to address issues that are likely to make a real difference to the well-being of patients. Chapter 7 maps what patients could do to ensure better testing of treatments. And in Chapter 8 we present our blueprint for a revolution in testing treatments – practical measures that could be started now to bring this about.

Each chapter is referenced with a key selection of source material; other sources of information are included in the Additional Resources section at the end of the book. For those who wish to explore issues in more detail, a good starting point is the James Lind Library at www.jameslindlibrary.org. This site also hosts an e-mail contact point for readers of *Testing Treatments* – do send us your comments to testingtreatments@jameslindlibrary.org.

Although we describe the harm that some inadequately tested treatments have caused, it is certainly not our intention to undermine patients' trust in their health professionals. Our aim is to improve communication and boost confidence. But this will only happen if patients can help their doctors critically assess treatment options. We hope that you, the reader, will emerge from this book sharing some of our passion for the subject and go on to ask awkward questions about treatments, identify gaps in medical knowledge, and get involved in research to find answers for the benefit of everybody.

1

NEW – BUT NO BETTER
OR EVEN WORSE

Virtually every week there seems to be a news story highlighting an unanticipated drug side-effect, a surgical mishap, a rampant infection, or a mismanaged pregnancy. Some critics go further: they portray today's science-based medicine as dehumanising – as if the butchery that preceded modern surgery or the poisons that once passed for therapeutic drugs were somehow more humane.[2]

Yet modern medicine has been hugely successful.[3] The development of effective drugs has revolutionised the treatment of heart attacks and high blood pressure and enabled many people with schizophrenia to emerge from mental hospitals to live at home. The effectiveness of drugs for stomach ulcers has done away with the need for major surgery, and futile treatments such as milk diets have been consigned to history. Childhood immunisation has made polio and diphtheria distant memories. It is easy to forget that leukaemia was once an almost uniformly fatal disease; and patients now regularly live with other cancers instead of dying from them. In west and equatorial Africa, the disease known as river blindness, which is caused by the larva of a type of fly, once left many people blind. It has now been virtually eradicated by drug treatment.

Modern imaging techniques have also brought significant benefits. Ultrasound, computed tomography (CT), and magnetic resonance imaging (MRI) have helped to ensure that patients are accurately diagnosed and receive the right treatment. For example, MRI can reveal what type of stroke a patient has suffered. If the stroke is caused by bleeding into the brain (haemorrhagic stroke), then aspirin, which is useful in other types of stroke, might be dangerous. Surgical and anaesthetic techniques, too, have

Sir Raymond Crawfurd (1865-1938) wrote a vivid account of the death of King Charles II in 1685. The King had suffered a stroke. His physicians rushed into action with an array of barbarous therapies:

'Sixteen ounces of blood were removed from a vein in his right arm with immediate good effect. As was the approved practice at this time, the King was allowed to remain in the chair in which the convulsions seized him. His teeth were held forcibly open to prevent him biting his tongue. The regimen was, as Roger North pithily describes it, first to get him to wake, and then to keep him from sleeping. Urgent messages had been dispatched to the King's numerous personal physicians, who quickly came flocking to his assistance; they were summoned regardless of distinctions of creed and politics, and they came. They ordered cupping-glasses to be applied to his shoulders forthwith, and deep scarification to be carried out, by which they succeeded in removing another eight ounces of blood. A strong antimonial emetic [a medicine to cause vomiting] was administered, but as the King could be got to swallow only a small portion of it, they determined to render assistance doubly sure by a full dose of Sulphate of Zinc. Strong purgatives were given, and supplemented by a succession of clysters [enemas]. The hair was shorn close, and pungent blistering agents were applied all over his head. And as though this were not enough, red-hot cautery was requisitioned as well. The King apologised for being "an unconscionable time a-dying".'

Crawfurd R. *Last days of Charles II.* Oxford: The Clarendon Press, 1909.

been greatly improved. Artificial joints have helped countless people, and organ transplants have become commonplace.

Of course many improvements in health have come about because of social and public health advances, such as piped clean water, sanitation, and better nutrition and housing. But even sceptics would be hard put to dismiss the impressive impact of modern medical care. Over the past half century, much of our increased life expectancy can be attributed to better healthcare, as can years of improved quality of life for those with chronic (persistent) diseases.[4]

Even now, however, too much medical decision-making is based on poor evidence and there are still too many medical treatments that harm patients, and worthwhile treatments that are not used enough (see below, and Chapter 5). Almost invariably there will be uncertainties about effects and effectiveness when new treatments are devised – treatment effects are very seldom overwhelmingly obvious. So, carefully designed fair tests are necessary to identify the effects reliably (see Chapter 3). Without a fair – unbiased – evaluation, the risk is that useless or even harmful treatments are deemed helpful or, conversely, that helpful treatments are dismissed as useless. Untested theories about treatments effects, however convincing they may sound, are not enough. Some theories have predicted that treatments would work, but actual evidence has revealed otherwise; other theories have confidently predicted that treatments would not work when, in fact, tests showed that they did.

There is nothing new in this: in the 18th century James Lind used a fair test to compare six of the remedies then being used to treat scurvy, a disease that was killing vast numbers of sailors during long voyages. He showed that (vitamin-C-containing) oranges and lemons were a very effective cure. In essence, Lind conducted what is now called a controlled trial.

In 1747, while serving as a ship's surgeon aboard HM 4th Rate Ship *Salisbury*, James Lind assembled 12 of his patients at similar stages of the illness, accommodated them in the same part of the ship, and ensured that they had the same basic diet. This was crucial – it creating a 'level playing field' (see Chapter 3, and Chapter 4, box on page 59). Lind then allocated two sailors to receive each of six treatments that were then in use for scurvy – cider, sulphuric acid, vinegar, seawater, nutmeg, or two oranges and a lemon. The fruit won hands down, and the Admiralty later ordered that lemon juice be supplied to all ships, with the result that the deadly disease had disappeared from the Royal Navy by the end of the 18th century. Of the treatments Lind compared, the Royal College of Physicians favoured sulphuric acid while the Admiralty favoured vinegar – Lind's fair test showed that both these authorities were wrong. And medical authority is not infrequently wrong (see below, and Chapters 2, 5, and 6).

Similar uncertainties about the effects of treatments are often highlighted today when doctors and other clinicians differ about the best approach for a particular condition (see Chapter 4). In addressing these uncertainties the public as well as doctors have an important part to play. It is in the overwhelming interest of patients as well as professionals that research on treatments should be rigorous. Just as doctors must be assured that their treatment recommendations are based on sound evidence, so patients need to demand that this happens. Only by creating this critical partnership can the public have confidence in all that modern medicine has to offer (see Chapter 7).

UNEXPECTED BAD EFFECTS

At one time, doctors were clearly uncertain whether pregnant women with previous miscarriages and stillbirths could be helped by a synthetic (non-natural) oestrogen called diethylstilboestrol (DES). Some of them prescribed it and some did not. DES became popular in the early 1950s and was thought to improve a malfunction of the placenta that was believed to cause these problems. Those who used it were encouraged by reports of women with previous miscarriages and stillbirths who had had a surviving child after DES treatment.

For example, one British obstetrician, consulted by a woman who had had two stillborn babies, prescribed the drug from early pregnancy on-wards. The pregnancy ended with the birth of a liveborn baby. Reasoning that the woman's 'natural' capacity for successful childbearing may have improved over this time, the obstetrician withheld DES during the woman's fourth pregnancy; the baby died in the womb from 'placental insufficiency'. So, during the woman's fifth and sixth pregnancies, the obstetrician and the woman were in no doubt that DES should again be given, and the pregnancies both ended with liveborn babies. Both the obstetrician and the woman concluded that DES was a useful drug. Unfortunately, this conclusion was never substantiated in the unbiased studies that were actually being conducted and reported during the years over which the woman was receiving care.[5]

Even worse, almost 20 years later, the mother of a young woman with a rare tumour of the vagina suggested that her daughter's cancer might be due to the DES she had been prescribed during her pregnancy.[6] Since then, numerous studies have shown a range of serious side-effects of DES in both men and women who, as fetuses, had been exposed to the hormone while in the womb, including not only an increased frequency of rare cancers but also abnormalities of the reproductive system.

By the time it was officially declared that DES should not be used in pregnancy, several million men and women had been exposed to the drug. Knowing what we know now, if doctors had known how to distinguish the most reliable research on DES available in the 1950s, many fewer would have prescribed it. What is more, DES was never actually proved to be effective for the condition for which it had been prescribed in the first place. Tragically, this lack of evidence of benefit was widely overlooked.[7]

Another chilling example of a medical treatment that did more harm than good is thalidomide.[8] This sleeping pill was introduced in the late 1950s as a safer alternative to the barbiturates that were regularly prescribed at that time; unlike barbiturates, overdoses of thalidomide did not lead to coma. Thalidomide was especially recommended for pregnant women, in whom it was also used to relieve morning sickness.

Then, at the beginning of the 1960s, obstetricians began to see cases of severely malformed arms and legs in newborn babies. This previously rare condition results in such extremely shortened limbs that the hands and feet seem to arise directly from the body. Doctors in Germany and Australia linked these infant malformations with the fact that the mothers had taken thalidomide in early pregnancy. And one of the German mothers of an affected baby had a crucial role in this discovery – she reported that she had experienced tingling and weakness of her hands and feet when she was taking the drug, which set doctors thinking.

At the end of 1961, the manufacturer withdrew thalidomide. Many years later, after public campaigns and legal action, the victims began to receive compensation. The toll of these devastating abnormalities was immense – across the 46 or so countries where thalidomide was prescribed (in some countries even sold over the counter), thousands of babies were affected. The thalidomide tragedy stunned doctors, the pharmaceutical industry, and patients, and led to an overhaul of the process of drug development and licensing worldwide.[9]

The drug practolol may not be nearly as well known as thalidomide but it, too, did immense harm. Practolol belongs to a group of drugs called beta-blockers, which are used to treat heart disease caused by poor blood supply to the heart and also to control irregularities in heart rhythm. When the first beta-blockers were introduced there were warnings that they

The Yellow Card scheme was launched in Britain in 1964 after the birth defects caused by thalidomide made it obvious that following up problems after a drug had been licensed was extremely important. Since then, 400,000 reports have been filed to the CSM [Committee on Safety of Medicines], a unit of the Department of Health that receives and analyses the results. Initially, only doctors could file the reports, but nurses, pharmacists, coroners, dentists, radiographers and optometrists have all been encouraged to sign and post the cards. And after a review of the scheme last year, patients and carers are now invited to report suspected adverse reactions under a pilot project launched last month at www.yellowcard.gov.uk. Not only can you file a report online, but you can also see what other people have filed. This gives a good idea about trends occurring in the use of a particular medicine, even though these are reports about yet-unproven suspicions.

McCartney M. Doctor's notes. *The Guardian*: Health, 2005, Feb 8, p9.

should not be used in patients with asthma because they worsened their breathing difficulties; they also tended to make patients depressed – 'beta-blocker blues'. When practolol was marketed, having been licensed after animal testing and brief clinical trials in patients, it was promoted as having a more specific action on the heart than its predecessors, and therefore being safer for asthmatic patients. It also caused less depression. All in all, it looked extremely promising.

But after four years, a constellation of side-effects known as the practolol syndrome became noticeable in some of the patients who had received the drug.[10] There were eye complications such as dry eyes from reduced tear secretion, conjunctivitis, and damage to the cornea leading to impaired vision. There were also reports of skin reactions, deafness, and a serious condition known as sclerosing peritonitis, in which the normally translucent lining of the abdomen turns into a mass of fibrous scar tissue that strangles the gut and other abdominal organs.

With hindsight, early on in the clinical use of practolol, patients had reported the eye symptoms to their GPs, but the doctors had not associated these with the drug. This delay in recognition took its toll – when the manufacturer withdrew practolol from use by GPs in 1975, it left at least 7,000 victims in its wake in the UK alone.

Thirty years on, drug-testing regulations have been tightened up considerably, so could this happen again? The chances are undoubtedly less, but even with the very best drug-testing practices there can be no absolute guarantee of safety. The practolol story provides a telling lesson that remains true today – patients' observations and clinical alertness remain vitally important in identifying unexpected drug reactions.[11]

HOPED-FOR EFFECTS THAT DON'T MATERIALISE

Do not imagine that only drugs can harm – advice can be lethal too. Most people have heard of the American childcare specialist Dr Benjamin Spock – his best-selling book *Baby and Child Care* became a bible for both professionals and parents. Yet in giving one of his pieces of well-meaning advice Dr Spock got things badly wrong. With seemingly irrefutable logic – and certainly a degree of authority – from the 1956 edition of his book onwards he argued: 'There are two disadvantages to a baby's sleeping on his back. If he vomits he's more likely to choke on the vomitus. Also he tends to keep his head turned towards the same side . . . this may flatten the side of the head . . . I think it is preferable to accustom a baby to sleeping on his stomach from the start.'

Placing babies to sleep on their front (prone) became standard practice in hospitals and was dutifully followed at home by millions of parents. But we now know that this practice – which was never rigorously evaluated – led to tens of thousands of avoidable cot deaths.[12] Although not all cot deaths can be blamed on this unfortunate advice, there was a dramatic decline in these deaths when the practice was abandoned and the opposite advice was promoted. When clear evidence of the harmful effects of the prone sleeping position emerged in the 1980s, doctors and the media started to warn of the dangers and the numbers of cot deaths began to fall dramatically. The message was later reinforced by concerted 'back to sleep' campaigns to remove once and for all the negative influence of Dr Spock's regrettable pronouncement.

Dr Spock's advice may have seemed logical, but it was based on untested theory. Examples of the dangers of doing this are not hard to find. After having a heart attack, some people develop heart rhythm abnormalities – arrhythmias. Those who do are more likely to die prematurely than those who don't. Since there are drugs that suppress these arrhythmias, it seemed logical to suppose that these drugs would also reduce the risk of premature death after heart attack. In fact, the drugs had exactly the opposite effect. The drugs had been tested in clinical trials, but only to see whether they reduced heart rhythm abnormalities. When the accumulated evidence from trials was first reviewed systematically in 1983, there was no evidence that these drugs reduced mortality.[13] However, the drugs continued to be used – and killed people – for nearly a

Advice to place infants to sleep on the front gathered momentum in the USA with the publication of the 1956 edition of *A Baby's First Year* by Dr Spock. Similar advice was adopted in Europe and Australasia about a decade later and was followed by a steep rise in the incidence of SIDS [Sudden Infant Death Syndrome] during the 1970s and 1980s and in the proportion of babies placed on the front. Had the evidence been reviewed systematically in 1970 it would have shown a three-fold increased risk of SIDS in babies placed on the front compared with any other position. However, few researchers would have been aware of these results even though the first summary was provided in 1988. It was not until the early 1990s, after SIDS incidence declined by about 70% in areas where researchers had reversed health advice, that national 'back to sleep' campaigns were launched. In the UK, this was 21 years after the first clear evidence of harm, at a cost of at least 11,000 avoidable infant deaths. In the USA, where sleeping on the front was more common for much longer, the death toll was much higher.

Adapted from Gilbert R, Salanti G, Harden M, See S.
Infant sleeping position and the sudden infant death syndrome: systematic review of observational studies and historical review of clinicians' recommendations from 1940-2000. *International Journal of Epidemiology* 2005;34:74-87.

decade. At the peak of their use in the late 1980s, one estimate is that they caused tens of thousands of premature deaths every year in the USA alone. They were killing more Americans every year than had been killed in action during the whole of the Vietnam war.[14] It later emerged that, for commercial reasons, the results of some trials suggesting that the drugs were lethal had never been reported.[15]

If it were possible to limit the amount of brain damage in patients who suffer a stroke, their chances of disability should be lessened. In the 1980s, a drug called nimodipine, which belongs to a group of drugs called calcium antagonists, was tested for this purpose in stroke patients, and some animal experiments gave encouraging results. The future looked bright for nimodipine when a clinical trial in stroke patients published in 1988 suggested a beneficial effect. However, the results of several more clinical trials of nimodipine and other calcium antagonist drugs proved conflicting. One possibility was that patients benefited only if the drugs were given early after the onset of a stroke, and a review of nimodipine trials seemed to confirm this. But when the accumulated evidence of clinical trials involving nearly 8,000 patients was reviewed systematically in 1999, no overall beneficial effect of the drugs was found, even if used early.[16] Since the use of nimodipine was apparently based on sound evidence, how had this come about? When, in the light of the results of research in patients, the findings from animal experiments were systematically reviewed for the first time,[17] it became clear that the animal findings were dubious at best. There had therefore been no convincing justification for carrying out trials in stroke patients in the first place (see Chapter 5).

In women going through the menopause, hormone replacement therapy (HRT) is very effective in reducing the distressing hot flushes that are commonly experienced, and there is some evidence that it may help to prevent osteoporosis. Gradually, more and more beneficial effects were claimed for HRT, including prevention of heart attacks and stroke. And millions of women, advised by their doctors, began using HRT for longer because of claims of these and other extra benefits. However, the basis of these claims was very shaky.

Take heart attacks alone. For over 20 years, women were told that HRT would reduce their risk of this serious condition – in fact the advice was based on the results of biased (unfair) studies (see above and Chapter 3, box on page 29). Then, in 1997, there was a warning that the advice might be wrong: researchers from Finland and the UK[18] reviewed, systematically, the results of well-conducted studies. They found that, far from reducing heart disease, HRT might actually increase it. Some prominent commentators dismissed this conclusion, but its tentative result has now been confirmed by two large unbiased trials. Had the effects of HRT been assessed properly when it was first introduced, women would not have been misinformed and many of them would not have died prematurely. To make matters worse, unbiased evidence now shows that HRT increases the risk of stroke and of developing breast cancer.[19]

Overall, HRT continues to be a valuable treatment for women with menopausal symptoms. However, it is tragic that it was so heavily promoted specifically as a way of reducing heart attacks and stroke. Although the increased risk of these serious conditions is modest, the total number of women affected is very large indeed because HRT has been so widely prescribed.

Even if inadequately assessed treatments do not kill or harm, they can waste money. Eczema is a distressing skin complaint affecting both children and adults. The skin lesions are both unsightly and very itchy. Although the use of steroid creams is effective in this condition, there were concerns about the side-effects of these treatments. In the early 1980s a natural plant oil extract – evening primrose oil – emerged as a possible alternative with few side-effects.[20] Evening primrose oil contains an essential fatty acid called gamma linolenic acid (GLA) and there were plausible reasons for using it. One suggestion, for example, was that in eczema the

In January 2004, a hysterectomy patient wrote this letter to *The Lancet:*

'In 1986 I had a hysterectomy because of fibroids. The surgeon also removed my ovaries and found that I had endometriosis as well. Because I was then only 45 years old and would have had an immediate menopause, I was put onto hormone replacement therapy (HRT). The first year I took conjugated oestrogens (Premarin), but from 1988 until 2001 I had oestrogen implants every 6 months, given to me privately by the surgeon who did the operation. I was always a little dubious about having the treatment, since I felt I just did not have control over things once the implant was done, and also after several years had many headaches. Apart from that I felt very fit.

However, my surgeon assured me that HRT had so many advantages and that it suited me, which I agreed with. As time went on, HRT was reported to have more and more benefits and was not just the cosmetic drug it seemed to have been used for in its early years. It was now good for the heart, osteoporosis, and part defence against strokes. Every time I visited my surgeon, he seemed to have more evidence about the advantages of taking HRT.

My surgeon retired in 2001 and I went to my National Health Service doctor. What a shock! He told me the exact opposite of my private surgeon – that it would be a good idea to come off HRT: it could increase the risk of heart disease, strokes, and breast cancer, and be the cause of headaches. I did have one more implant and then went onto Premarin for a short while, but since then I have not used HRT for about 8 months. My doctor said it would be my decision whether to stay on it or not. I was so confused . . .

I cannot understand how HRT and all its wonderful advantages can be reversed in such a short space of time. How can a layman like myself come to a clear decision? I have spent many hours discussing and thinking about whether I should have stayed on HRT, although so far I have not suffered many ill effects. I am very confused about the whole issue and I am sure other women feel the same.'

Huntingford CA. Confusion over benefits
of hormone replacement therapy. *Lancet* 2004;363:332.

way in which GLA was transformed within the body (metabolised) was impaired. So, theoretically, giving GLA supplements would help. Borage oil, also known as starflower oil, contains even higher amounts of GLA and this was also recommended for eczema.

GLA was found to be safe but was it effective? Numerous studies were done to find out but they gave conflicting results. And the published evidence was heavily influenced by studies sponsored by the companies making the supplements. In 1995, the Department of Health requested researchers unconnected with the manufacturers of evening primrose oil to review 20 published and unpublished studies. No evidence of benefit was found. The Department never made the report public because the manufacturers of the drug objected. But five years later another review of both evening primrose oil and borage oil by the same researchers – this time it was published – showed that in the largest and most complete studies there was no convincing evidence that these treatments worked.[21]

There was one unturned stone – perhaps GLA only worked in very high doses. In 2003, even this claim was knocked on the head by a carefully conducted fair test.[22] Ironically, by the time these results were published, the Medicines Control Agency had finally, in October 2002, withdrawn the product licence for evening primrose oil – an expensive drug – because there was no evidence that the drug was useful.

It is equally important not to be dazzled by claims of success for the latest high-tech fix for a life-threatening disease. Severe infection with certain bacteria can lead to a very serious complication known as septic shock. This usually occurs in people with an underlying illness, or in those whose immune system is not functioning properly. In patients with septic shock, the blood pressure falls to dangerously low levels and the body's major organs fail. Despite intensive treatment for the infection, as many as four out of five patients may die.[23]

Although exactly how bacteria cause septic shock is still unclear, scientific insights beginning in the 1980s led to a theory that linked malfunction of the immune system with the condition. Most serious bacterial infections are caused by gram-negative bacteria (this refers to a standard method of classifying bacteria). Gram-negative bacteria are especially known to cause septic shock, although gram-positive bacteria sometimes do so as well. Gram-negative bacteria cause septic shock by releasing toxic substances called endotoxins into the bloodstream, and these stimulate cells to release other substances called cytokines. The cytokines damage the walls of capillaries, the small blood vessels that criss-cross the body, causing them to leak and so leading to shock and the fall in blood pressure.

Reasoning that the effects of septic shock should be lessened if it were possible to rid the blood of the damaging endotoxins and cytokines, scientists used the latest biotechnology to make antibodies specifically to neutralise the effects of endotoxin. These antibodies were first tested in animals, with encouraging results: gram-negative shock could be prevented provided the antibodies were given very early in the course of infection. However, the difficulty doctors face when a patient presents with septic shock is that it is impossible, straightaway, to say whether gram-negative or gram-positive bacteria are involved. Getting test results can take up to 72 hours. Nevertheless, the results of the first unbiased (fair) trial in patients were reported as a success.[24]

But doubts soon started to creep in. On closer inspection it became clear that the results had not been interpreted correctly. Subsequent clinical trials of tailor-made antibodies failed to show any benefit and sometimes even showed a small harmful effect. These consistently negative findings in unbiased studies challenged the scientific theory about the immune system in septic shock, showing that the relationship between endotoxins, cytokines, and septic shock was far more complex than originally imagined. Not surprisingly, the initial enthusiasm for use of the antibodies waned.

KEY POINTS

■ Biased (unfair) studies can lead to avoidable illness and premature deaths

■ Neither theory nor professional opinion by itself is a reliable guide to safe, effective treatments

■ Systematic reviews of studies are essential for designing and understanding both human and animal experiments

■ Patients can draw attention to unexpected effects of treatments

2

USED BUT INADEQUATELY TESTED

In Chapter 1 we learned that some new treatments have had harmful effects that were unexpected; the hoped-for effects of others failed to materialise; and some predictions that treatments would not work were proved wrong. This chapter highlights how commonly used treatments may not have been tested adequately. How can this happen? The therapies advocated for breast cancer – which are often in the news – provide some especially valuable lessons.

WHEN MORE IS NOT NECESSARILY BETTER

Throughout the 20th century and even into the 21st, women with breast cancer have endured some exceedingly brutal and distressing treatments. These treatments – both surgical and medical – far exceeded what was actually required to tackle the disease. But they were also unquestionably popular with some patients as well as their doctors. Patients were convinced that the more radical or toxic the therapy, the more likely the disease would be conquered. It took courageous doctors and outspoken patient advocates many years to begin to turn the tide of misbelief. They not only had to produce reliable evidence to banish the myth that 'more is better', but also suffer the ridicule of their peers and the resistance of eminent practitioners.

Even today, fear, coupled with the belief that more must be better, drives treatment choices. This prompts some patients and their doctors to opt for 'traditional' mutilating and painful treatments, for which there is no evidence of benefit over simpler approaches. How can this be?

'It is very easy for those of us treating cancer to imagine that better results are due to a more drastic treatment. Randomized trials comparing drastic treatment with less drastic treatment are vital in order to protect patients from needless risk and the early or late side effects of unnecessarily aggressive treatment. The comparison is ethical because those who are denied possible benefit are also shielded from possible unnecessary harm – and nobody knows which it will turn out to be in the end.'

Rees G, ed. *The friendly professional: selected writings of Thurstan Brewin.* Bognor Regis: Eurocommunica, 1996.

Until the middle of the 20th century, surgery was the main treatment for breast cancer. This was based on the belief that the cancer progressed in a slow and orderly manner, in the first instance from the tumour site in the breast to local lymph nodes, in the armpit, for example. Consequently it was reasoned that the more radical and prompt the surgery for the tumour, the better the chance of halting the spread of the cancer. Treatment was essentially by extensive 'local' surgery – that is, surgery on or near the breast. It may have been called local, but a radical mastectomy was anything but – it involved removing large areas of chest muscle and much lymph node tissue from the armpits.

However, some thoughtful and observant breast cancer specialists noted that these increasingly mutilating operations did not seem to be having any impact on death rates from breast cancer. So, they put forward a different theory – that breast cancer, rather than spreading from the breast in an orderly manner through the nearby lymph nodes, was in fact a systemic disease from the outset. In other words, they reasoned that cancer cells must already be present elsewhere in the body at the time the breast lump was detected. If so, they suggested, removal of the tumour with an adequate margin of normal tissue, plus a course of radiotherapy, would be both kinder to the woman and might be as effective as radical treatment. The introduction of 'systemic therapies' at about this time – that is, treatments that would deal with production or development of cancer cells elsewhere in the body – was also based on this new theory of breast cancer spread.

As a direct result of this new way of thinking, doctors advocated more limited surgery known as lumpectomy – that is, removal of the tumour and a margin of surrounding normal tissue – which was followed by radiotherapy, and in some women by chemotherapy. But they encountered

The radical mastectomy, devised in the late 19th century by Sir William Halsted, was the most commonly performed operation for breast cancer until the third quarter of the 20th century. As well as removing all of the breast, the surgeon cut away the pectoralis major muscle covering the chest wall. The smaller pectoralis minor muscle was also removed to allow the surgeon easier access to the armpit (axilla) to clear out the lymph nodes and surrounding fat.

EXTENDED RADICAL MASTECTOMIES

During that time, the belief that 'more is better' led radical surgeons to carry out even more extensive operations, in which chains of lymph nodes under the collarbone and the internal mammary nodes under the breastbone were also removed. To get at the internal mammary nodes several ribs were removed and the breastbone was split with a chisel. Not content with that, some surgeons went so far as to remove the arm on the affected side and cut out various glands throughout the body (adrenals, pituitary, ovaries) to suppress the production of hormones that were believed to 'fuel' the spread of the tumour.

If a woman survived such operations she was left with a severely mutilated ribcage, which was difficult to conceal under any clothing. If surgery had been carried out on the left side, only a thin layer of skin remained to cover the heart.

Adapted from Lerner BH, *The breast cancer wars: hope, fear and the pursuit of a cure in twentieth-century America.* New York: Oxford University Press, 2003.

huge resistance to comparing the new approach with radical surgery. Some doctors believed very firmly in one or other approach and patients clamoured for one or other treatment. The result was a massive delay in producing the crucial evidence about the merits and harms of the proposed new treatment compared with the old.

Nevertheless, despite these difficulties, the surgical excesses were eventually challenged, both by surgeons who were unwilling to continue in the face of questionable benefits for their patients, and by outspoken women who were unwilling to undergo mutilating operations.

In the mid-1950s, George Crile, an American surgeon, led the way by going public with his concerns about the 'more is better' approach. Believing that there was no other tactic to stir doctors into thinking critically, Crile appealed to them in an article in *Life* magazine.[25] He hit the right note: the debate within the medical profession was now out in the open, and in full public view. Then another US surgeon, Bernard Fisher, working together with colleagues in other specialties, devised a series of rigorous experiments to study the biology of cancer. Their results suggested that cancer cells could indeed travel widely through the blood stream, even before the primary cancer was discovered. So, increasingly aggressive surgery made little sense if the cancer was already present elsewhere in the body.

Whereas Crile had used his clinical judgment to advocate and employ less radical local therapies, Fisher and a growing group of researchers collaborated in a more formal and rigorous approach. They sought to prove or disprove the value of radical surgery by the best-known unbiased (fair) method – randomised controlled trials (see Chapter 3). They reasoned that by doing such studies the medical community and the general public might be convinced one way or the other. In 1971, the outspoken Fisher also declared that surgeons had an ethical and moral responsibility to test their theories by conducting such trials. And certainly, the 20-year follow-up of Fisher's trials showed that – as measured by the risk of early death – breast cancer could be treated as effectively by lumpectomy followed by radiation therapy as by total mastectomy.[26]

Meanwhile, in the UK, the first randomised controlled trial (see Chapter 3, and Chapter 4, box on page 59) comparing breast-conserving therapy with classical radical mastectomy was conducted by Hedley Atkins and colleagues at Guy's Hospital early in the 1960s. Similarly, this showed that there was little difference in outcomes between the two treatments in the 20 years after diagnosis. Other randomised trials, in Sweden and Italy as well as the UK and the USA, were done to compare many other forms of treatment – for example, radiation therapy after surgery compared with surgery alone, and short-term compared with long-term chemotherapies.

By 1985, the sheer volume of breast cancer trials made it very difficult for doctors to keep sufficiently up to date with all the results. To address this problem, Richard Peto and his colleagues in Oxford drew together all the trial findings in the first systematic review (see Chapter 3) of all the information about all of the women who had participated in the many studies.[27] Cancer specialists and the general public could then access the latest amalgamated worldwide evidence. Systematic reviews of treatments for breast cancer are now updated and published regularly.

However, the demise of mutilating surgery did not spell the end of the 'more is better' mindset – far from it. During the last two decades of the 20th century, a treatment approach involving high-dose chemotherapy followed by bone marrow transplantation or 'stem cell rescue' held considerable sway. A critical special report in the *New York Times* in 1999 summed up the reasoning behind this approach:

> 'Doctors remove some bone marrow or red blood cells from the patient, then load her with huge amounts of toxic drugs, quantities that destroy the bone marrow. The hope is that the high doses will eliminate the cancer and that the saved bone marrow, when returned to the body, will grow back quickly enough so that the patient does not die from infection. A version of the procedure, using donations of bone marrow, had long been established as effective for blood cancer, but solely because the cancer was in the marrow that was being replaced. The use of the treatment for breast cancer involved a completely different – and untested – reasoning.'[28]

In the USA especially, thousands of desperate women asked for this very unpleasant treatment from doctors and hospitals who were only too willing to provide it. As many as five out of 100 patients died from the treatment. Thousands of dollars were spent, some of this money coming from the patients' own pockets. Eventually, some patients were reimbursed by their health insurance companies, who caved in to pressure to do so, despite the lack of evidence. Many hospitals and clinics became rich on the proceeds. In 1998, one hospital corporation brought in $128 million in revenue, largely from its cancer centres providing bone marrow transplants. For US doctors it was a lucrative source of income and prestige and it provided a rich field for producing publications. Insistent patient demand fuelled the market. Competition from private US hospitals to provide the

---

THE STRUGGLE FOR UNBIASED EVIDENCE

Researchers expected it would take about three years to enrol about 1,000 women in the two studies. Instead it took seven years . . . That is not so surprising . . . Patients in the clinical trials must sign a consent form spelling out their grim prognosis and stating that there is no evidence that bone marrow transplants are any better than standard therapies. To enter the trial, you have to face these realities, which is never easy. But if the patient has a transplant outside a trial with a control group of patients, known as a randomised trial, enthusiastic doctors may tell her that a transplant could save her life. Although patients have a right to the truth, they understandably are not going to go to doctors who take away hope.

Adapted from Kolata G, Eichenwald K. Health business thrives on unproven treatment, leaving science behind. *New York Times* Special Report, 1999, 2 October.

---

treatments was intense, with cut-price offers advertised. In the 1990s, even US academic medical centres trying to recruit patients for clinical trials were offering this treatment. These questionable programmes had become the 'cash cow' for the cancer services.

Unrestricted access to such non-proven treatments had another serious downside: there were not enough patients available to take part in trials comparing these treatments with standard therapies. As a result it took far longer than anticipated to get reliable answers.

But despite the difficulties of obtaining unbiased evidence in the face of such pressures, some clinical trials were carried out and other evidence reviewed critically. And in 2004, a systematic review of the accumulated results of high-dose chemotherapy followed by bone marrow transplantation, as a general treatment for breast cancer, revealed no convincing evidence that it was useful.[29, 30]

SCREENING APPARENTLY WELL PEOPLE FOR EARLY SIGNS OF ILLNESS

Screening apparently well people for early signs of illness sounds so sensible – how better to ward off serious consequences of disease and stay healthy? Already several disorders, especially cancers, are the target of national screening programmes, and numerous private clinics promote regular health checks – essentially a battery of screening tests – claiming that these will help their clients stay well. Yet while some screening tests are helpful – measuring blood pressure, for example – others may be harmful.

So, before rushing headlong into widespread screening, it is worth pausing a moment to consider what screening aims to achieve. The main

---

FROM PERSON TO PATIENT

Screening will inevitably turn some people who test 'positive' into patients – a transformation not to be undertaken lightly. 'If a patient asks a medical practitioner for help, the doctor does the best possible. The doctor is not responsible for defects in medical knowledge. If, however, the practitioner initiates screening procedures the doctor is in a very different situation. The doctor should, in our view, have conclusive evidence that screening can alter the natural history of the disease in a significant proportion of those screened.'

Cochrane AL, Holland WW. Validation of screening procedures.
British Medical Bulletin 1971;27:3-8.

aim of screening individuals or populations is to reduce the risk of death or serious disability in a specific disease by offering a test intended to help identify people who could benefit from treatment.[31] The basic criteria for assessing the value of screening tests were outlined in a World Health Organisation report in 1968 and are still worth remembering:

- The condition sought should pose an important health problem
- There should be an effective and acceptable treatment for the condition
- There should be adequate facilities for the diagnosis and treatment of abnormalities detected
- There should be a recognisable early stage of the condition
- There should be a valid test
- The test should be acceptable to the population
- The natural history of the condition should be adequately understood
- The chance of physical or psychological harm to those screened should be less than the chance of benefit
- Screening should be a continuing process and not a once and for all project
- The screening programme should be cost-effective.[32]

Today, with the benefit of hindsight, one can identify three important shortcomings in these principles. First, the harmful effects of screening are not emphasised sufficiently. Few tests, if any, are risk free – in the sense that they are imperfect in their ability to pinpoint the disease in question. For example, they may not detect all or most of the people with the condition – they are not sensitive enough. Or they may overdiagnose the condition – they are not specific enough. And, when people have been given a disease label, they often find themselves on a roller coaster of further tests, associated anxieties, and sometimes unjustified discrimination, for example by insurance companies. Second, the criteria emphasise that there should be an effective and acceptable treatment for the disease – yet many currently accepted treatments are of unproven value. And the recommended treatments based on the results of these imperfect screening tests inevitably carry their own risks. Third, the criteria do not emphasise that the decision to introduce a screening programme should be based on good quality evidence.[33]

What lessons can one learn from current screening programmes? Experience with screening for neuroblastoma – a rare malignant tumour that affects predominantly young children – is instructive. It was a tempting target for screening for four reasons: (1) children who are diagnosed before the age of one year are known to have a better outlook than those who are diagnosed later; (2) children with advanced disease fare much worse than those with early disease; (3) there is a simple and cheap screening test that can be carried out by blotting wet nappies and measuring a substance in the urine; and (4) the test detects nine out of 10 children with neuroblastoma.[34]

Mass screening for neuroblastoma was first introduced in Japan in the 1980s, but 20 years later there was no evidence that neuroblastoma screening had reduced the chance of death from this cancer. Screening was started in Japan without the benefit of unbiased (fair) evidence from clinical trials. By contrast, clinical trials done in Canada and Germany, involving about three million children in all, suggested that there was no obvious benefit of screening but there were obvious harms.[35] The harms included unjustified surgery and chemotherapy, both of which can have serious unwanted effects. A specialist, commenting on the Canadian and German results, didn't mince words:

'Screening for neuroblastoma illustrates how easily one can fall into the trap of assuming that because a disease can be detected early, screening must be worthwhile . . . The two studies demonstrate how neuroblastoma screening was not only worthless, but led to "over-diagnosis" and must have identified tumours that would have spontaneously regressed. Both studies mentioned children in the screened group suffering severe complications due to the treatment . . . Hopefully these lessons will be learned when considering the implementation of other screening programmes – for example screening for prostate cancer.'[36]

Prostate cancer is very different from neuroblastoma – it is a common cancer, which affects adult men. (In England and Wales it is the second most common cancer in men.[37]) Yet the same principles of screening

'People will value benefits and harms of screening differently. For example, pregnant women who are considering screening for Down syndrome may make different choices depending on the value they place on having a Down syndrome baby vs the risk of iatrogenic [caused inadvertently by the doctor] abortion from amniocentesis.

Individuals who choose to participate in screening programs are benefiting (in their view) from screening, and other individuals are benefiting (in their view) from not participating. Individuals can only make the right choice for themselves if they have access to high-quality information about the benefits and harms of screening and are able to weigh that information.'

Barratt A, Irwig L, Glasziou P, *et al*. Users' guides to the medical literature. XVII. How to use guidelines and recommendations about screening. *Journal of the American Medical Association* 1999;281:2029-33.

should apply. So how does prostate cancer screening measure up? A raised blood level of a substance called prostate-specific antigen (PSA) is associated with an increased risk of death from prostate cancer. But there are no published unbiased (fair) trials showing that earlier detection improves a man's outcome.[38] However, it is clear that PSA testing can cause harm. Some men will be treated when their cancers are too advanced to be helped; others will be treated unnecessarily when they have the sort of prostate cancer that would never pose a danger to health or life. In both groups of men, the treatment carried out as a result of a raised PSA measurement can cause distressing side-effects such as incontinence and impotence.

Yet in the USA and Italy, for example, at least a third of healthy men aged over 50 years have had PSA measured. The pro-PSA lobby in the USA – and that includes the public and patients as well as doctors – is especially powerful. In 2001, the *San Francisco Chronicle* published an article about the manager of the city's baseball team. He had just had prostate cancer surgery after the result of a routine PSA test came back 'positive'. The article presented PSA screening in a very favourable light; the drawbacks were not mentioned. Seeking to redress the balance before the *Chronicle*'s male readers took a wholly optimistic view of PSA screening, two doctors contacted the newspaper arguing that the article did not reflect the massive controversy surrounding PSA screening. They were invited to write a piece discussing the reasons why men should not be screened.

This article unleashed an extraordinary response. Within hours of

In 1999, a doctor training in family (general) practice in the USA saw a 53-year-old man for a physical examination. He discussed with him, and documented in the patient's notes, the importance of colon cancer screening, seat belts, dental care, exercise, improved diet, and sunscreen use. He also presented the risks of, and benefits for, prostate cancer screening. He never saw the patient again.

As it happened the man went to see a second doctor, who ordered PSA testing without discussing the possible benefits and risks of screening. The PSA result came back very high and the man was subsequently found to have incurable advanced prostate cancer. Although there is no evidence that early detection would have changed the man's outcome, the patient sued the first doctor and that doctor's family practice training programme.

The doctor's own words tell the rest of the story: 'Although we had the recommendations from every nationally recognized group supporting my approach and the literature is clear that screening for prostate cancer is controversial, the plaintiff's attorney argued otherwise . . . A major part of the plaintiff's case was that I did not practice the standard of care in the Commonwealth of Virginia. Four physicians testified that when they see male patients older than 50 years, they have no discussion with the patient about prostate cancer screening: they simply do the test. This was a very cogent argument, since in all likelihood more than 50% of physicians do practice in this way. One may have argued that we were practicing above the standard of care, but there is no legal precedent for such an argument . . . seven days after the trial started, I was exonerated. My residency [training programme] was found liable for $1 million . . . As I see it, the only way to practice medicine is to keep up with the best available evidence and bring it to my patients. As I see it, the only way to see patients is by using the shared decision-making model. As I see it, the only way to step into an examination room is to look at a patient as a whole person, not as a potential plaintiff. As I see it, I'm not sure I'll ever want to practice again.'

Merenstein D. Winners and losers.
Journal of the American Medical Association 2004;291:15-16.

publication, prostate cancer charities, patient support groups, and urologists had responded in force. The doctors who had written the article were showered with abuse by e-mail, compared with the Nazi doctor Mengele, and accused of having the deaths of hundreds of thousands of men on their hands. They wondered why they had provoked this fierce backlash, and wrote: 'One reason is that the PSA advocacy group is passionate in its belief that routine testing is good for men's health. It wishes to believe that screening really does make "a world of difference". We angered this group by challenging its wishful thinking. We also stepped on the toes of a very wealthy and powerful pro-screening lobby that stands to make money from encouraging men to get tested. Even some of the patient support groups have a conflict of interest, since they rely on pharmaceutical company support.'[39]

What about screening newborn babies for cystic fibrosis? This life-threatening disease usually produces symptoms from early childhood. Among other complications, it leads to chronic and debilitating chest infections with eventual permanent lung damage, failure to absorb food, stunted growth, and liver failure. Cystic fibrosis is a genetic condition, usually arising when the children have two disease-forming mutations in a gene. Those with one gene mutation are carriers of the condition but do

---

CYSTIC FIBROSIS SCREENING IN NEWBORN BABIES

BENEFITS

- To provide each family with a cystic fibrosis infant the opportunity of specialist care
- Reduction in the distress associated with delayed diagnosis
- Potential for all cystic fibrosis cases to be included on a national database
- Opportunity to carry out large randomised controlled trials of treatments

RISKS

- There is no perfect screening test for cystic fibrosis in newborn babies – cases will be missed and doctors will need to remain vigilant to the possible diagnosis in adults
- Identification of carrier status may result in distress
- Families may still be upset if the result of screening is not given in a thoughtful and empathetic manner
- Parents of 'well' children with cystic fibrosis will still find the situation stressful (in some ways it is more difficult to be living with the anticipation of future deterioration in the condition)

Southern KW. Newborn screening for cystic fibrosis: the practical implications. *Journal of the Royal Society of Medicine* 2004;97(suppl 44):57-9.

not have the symptoms themselves. Except that it is not quite that simple – the more that is discovered about the genetic basis of cystic fibrosis, the more complexities are revealed. Numerous 'atypical' types of cystic fibrosis are now known to exist.[40]

Over the years, the life expectancy of people with cystic fibrosis has undoubtedly advanced substantially as physiotherapy, antibiotics, and nutritional supplements have been used more intensively. In theory, early diagnosis by means of screening should have much to offer, especially before the lungs become seriously damaged. Although there is no universal agreement about the best combination of screening tests, newborn screening has already been introduced in several countries.

On the benefit side, infants diagnosed early by screening are more likely to achieve normal height and weight than those diagnosed later when they have symptoms.[41] However, any effect on preventing lung damage is far less certain. And the drawbacks of identifying babies who are cystic fibrosis gene carriers should not be underestimated. There will be implications later in life if carriers choose to have children of their own, and more immediately there are implications for relatives who may be similarly affected. As two researchers put it: 'Screening provides an opportunity to achieve good results but does not automatically guarantee a good outcome'.[42]

DRAWBACKS OF IDENTIFYING CYSTIC FIBROSIS GENE CARRIERS

'Although the family may be relieved to hear that the child is not affected by cystic fibrosis, there is concern that anxiety and grief reactions associated with the carrier state diagnosis may place families at risk for impaired parent-child bonding, personality problems, disrupted relationships or some variant of the vulnerable child syndrome. Other potential drawbacks to the identification of carriers are the recognition of non-paternity (and subsequent family break-up), stigmatisation of the child, difficulties with medical or life insurance and employment discrimination (due to a misconception about the potential harm of carrier status), and devaluing of a child as a potential marriage partner. Finally, if an infant's cystic fibrosis gene mutation is not included in the standard cystic fibrosis gene screening panel there is a risk that a negative screening result will be falsely reassuring.'

David TJ. Newborn screening for cystic fibrosis.
Journal of the Royal Society of Medicine 2004;97:209-10.

IS IT WISE TO SCREEN FOR IMPACTED WISDOM TEETH?

One of the most regular screening programmes is routine dental check-ups. Yet there has been evidence for several years that they may do more harm than good. One way they can do this is by leading to the removal of wisdom teeth. Wisdom teeth are the last permanent teeth to appear, usually between 18 and 24 years of age. Sometimes, however, they become impacted – that is, they fail to emerge from the gums – for various reasons. In most cases impacted wisdom teeth do not cause any problems, but some people do get complications such as inflammation of the surrounding gum and decay of surrounding teeth and bone. Although removal of impacted wisdom teeth that are causing problems is uncontroversial, removal of impacted teeth that are healthy is a different matter. And removal of these teeth is also painful and costly – in England and Wales alone, the NHS has spent millions of pounds on this type of dental surgery. So, the National Institute for Health and Clinical Excellence (NICE), which is charged with looking at evidence impartially and issuing advice, was asked to investigate the issue and guide the NHS. After reviewing the evidence, its conclusion, published in 2000, was categorical: impacted wisdom teeth that are free from disease should not be operated on. NICE gave two reasons for its conclusion: (a) there is no reliable research to suggest that this practice benefits patients; and (b) patients who do have healthy wisdom teeth removed are being exposed to the risks of surgery. These can include nerve damage, damage to other teeth, infection, bleeding and, rarely, death. Also, after surgery to remove wisdom teeth, patients may have swelling and pain and be unable to open their mouth fully.[43]

AND SO TO BED

We have seen how over-treatment and over-zealous screening can do more harm than good, yet even recommending something as apparently harmless as bed rest can be misguided. Bed rest is often assumed to be good for most illnesses. Nevertheless, if it is prescribed as a treatment to speed recovery – and it has been for a wide range of conditions, and after surgery – the benefits and harms should be assessed critically as for any other therapy. Doubts about the value of bed rest first emerged in the 1940s, when studies in patients after surgical operations showed no advantages for complete bed rest and suggested instead that there were potential dangers such as blood clots in the legs and bedsores. So, what is the unbiased evidence, if any, for benefit or harm of bed rest as a treatment? In 1999, researchers in Australia decided to review, systematically, the published unbiased (fair) assessments of bed rest as a treatment to find out whether there was any evidence of benefit or harm.[44] They found a total of 39 clinical trials of bed rest in 15 different conditions, in all involving nearly 6,000 patients, and looked for several possible effects of treatment – good and bad.

There were two main uses of bed rest as a treatment: first as a preventive measure after a medical or surgical procedure, and second as a first-line (primary) treatment. In 24 controlled trials of bed rest following a procedure no clear benefits were detected. In nine studies bed rest made matters worse after some procedures, including bed rest after lumbar puncture and spinal anaesthesia. In 15 trials of bed rest as a first-line treatment for various conditions, again there were no clear benefits. And in nine trials there was evidence of harm for some conditions, including low back pain, childbirth, and heart attacks. Overall, the evidence of the effects of bed rest in the conditions in which it has been studied suggests that it may actually delay recovery and even be harmful.

KEY POINTS

- More intensive treatment is not necessarily beneficial
- Looking for disease in apparently healthy people can do more harm than good

3

KEY CONCEPTS
IN FAIR TESTS
OF TREATMENTS

In the first two chapters we have shown how treatments that are inadequately tested can cause serious harm. Clearly it is vital that treatments are tested rigorously to help decide whether they should be offered to patients.

Misleading claims about treatments are common, so all of us need to be able to decide whether claims about the effects of treatments are valid. Without this knowledge, we risk concluding that useless treatments are helpful, or that helpful treatments are useless. To test treatments fairly, steps must be taken to obtain reliable information about treatment effects. Most importantly, the distorting influence of biases and the play of chance must be reduced. How should this be done?

REMOVING RUBBISH ON THE WAY TO KNOWLEDGE

When James Lind (see Chapter 1) began to read the literature on scurvy, he realised that the only existing descriptions of the disease were by lay seamen and by doctors who had never been to sea. 'No physician conversant with this disease at sea had undertaken to throw light upon the subject.' Lind felt that this was one of the reasons why there was so much confusion about the diagnosis, prevention and cure of the disease. As Lind wrote bluntly: 'Indeed, before the subject could be set in clear and proper light, it was necessary to remove a great deal of rubbish.'

Lind J. *A treatise of the scurvy. In three parts. Containing an inquiry into the nature, causes and cure, of that disease. Together with a critical and chronological view of what has been published on the subject.* Edinburgh: Printed by Sands, Murray and Cochran for A Kincaid and A Donaldson, 1753, pviii.

Biases in tests of treatment are those influences and factors that can lead to conclusions about treatment effects that differ from the truth systematically, and not just by chance. Although many kinds of biases can distort the results of health research, the biases that must be minimised in fair tests of treatments are:

- biases due to differences in people compared;
- biases due to differences in the way treatment effects are assessed;
- biased reporting of the available evidence; and
- biased selection from the available evidence

The principles we cover here will not be familiar to many of you, and some readers will find this chapter the most challenging in the book. Fuller information and illustrations about the key issues are contained in The James Lind Library (www.jameslindlibrary.org), and we hope that you will find the additional material there helpful.

FAIR TESTS OF MEDICAL TREATMENTS

Comparisons are the key to all fair tests of treatments; they are essential for judging whether or not a treatment causes a certain effect. Sometimes two or more treatments are compared; or a treatment is compared with no active treatment. Whatever the comparison, it should address a genuine uncertainty about treatment effects – that is, there is no convincing evidence from research. (We introduced the concept of uncertainty in Chapter 1 and we describe how to deal with it in chapter 4.) And for comparisons to be fair they must be as unbiased as possible.

Why comparisons are essential

The need for comparisons of treatments is easy to understand if one pauses to think for a moment. The old adage that Nature is a great healer happens to be true – people often recover from illness without any specific treatment at all. So, the 'natural' progress and outcome of illness without treatment must be taken into account when treatments are being tested. The treatment may improve – or worsen – the outcome that would have occurred naturally – or have nothing to do with the outcome at all.

People – clinicians and patients alike – sometimes make mental comparisons about the effects of treatments. They form an impression that they or others are responding differently to a new treatment than they did to earlier treatments. These impressions need to be followed up by formal investigations – for example, initially by analysis of clinical records. Such analyses may then lead to carefully conducted comparisons of new and old treatments.

The danger arises when impressions alone are used to guide treatment recommendations (see Chapter 1, page 4). Treatment comparisons based on impressions or initial analyses are seldom reliable. Only when treatment effects are dramatic – for example, the use of opium for relief of pain, insulin for diabetes, or hip replacements for osteoarthritis – will this be so (see Chapter 4). In most cases, however, treatment effects are more modest and precautions are needed to avoid biased comparisons and mistaken conclusions.

Comparisons of treatments given today with those given in the past are often unreliable because other relevant factors will have changed over time. One of the examples we cited in Chapter 1 – use of the hormone diethylstilboestrol (DES) to prevent recurrent stillbirths – illustrates this point well. Stillbirths are more common in first pregnancies than in subsequent ones. So, comparisons of stillbirth rates during second and subsequent pregnancies in which DES was prescribed with rates in first pregnancies in which it was not prescribed gave seriously misleading results, suggesting that DES reduced the risk of stillbirth. And in this example, as we showed, there were grave consequences for some of the children whose mothers were given the drug. Whenever possible, therefore, comparisons should be of different treatments given more or less at the same time.

Why comparisons must address genuine uncertainties

Before embarking on new tests of treatments it is essential to establish what is already known. Although this seems obvious, many uncertainties about the effects of treatments have come about because existing reliable evidence was ignored. Such evidence needs to be reviewed systematically and critically to be sure that the proposed new test of treatment will address a genuine current uncertainty. If this key preliminary step is overlooked, the consequences can be serious – patients have suffered unnecessarily, and precious healthcare and research resources have been squandered. How is this possible?

In the early 1990s, a team of researchers in the USA looked in medical textbooks and journals to identify the recommendations for the treatment of heart attacks made over a period of 30 years.[45] They then compared these recommendations with the evidence that could have been taken into account had the results of fair tests been reviewed systematically. The researchers found that, because the authors of the textbooks had not bothered to reduce the misleading effects of bias and the play of chance when they reviewed the evidence, there were serious consequences for patients. In some cases patients had been deprived of reliable advice on life-saving therapies (for example, clot-busting drugs for heart attacks), sometimes for more than a decade; in others, doctors had continued to recommend treatments long after fair tests had shown they were harmful (for example, anti-arrhythmic drugs in heart attack – see Chapter 1).

Researchers who do not review past tests of treatments before embarking on new studies may not realise that uncertainties about treatment effects have already been convincingly addressed. This means that some patients are taking part in research unnecessarily and being denied treatment that can help them. For example, long after there was reliable evidence that giving antibiotics to patients having bowel surgery reduced their chances of dying from complications of the operation, researchers continued to do comparison studies that involved withholding antibiotics from half the patients participating in the studies (see Chapter 5). Conversely, sometimes when previous results are reviewed it soon becomes apparent that reliable evidence is lacking – so new studies are definitely needed.

And, as we pointed out in Chapter 1 (page 9), patients can also suffer when researchers have not reviewed relevant evidence from animal research systematically before beginning to test treatments in patients. In that example, had the results of animal experiments been reviewed, clinical trials of the drug nimodipine in stroke patients would never have been done.

The idea of reviewing evidence systematically is far from new. The subtitle of James Lind's 1753 *Treatise of the Scurvy*, in which he reported his fair test of then favoured remedies (see Chapter 1), indicates that it contains 'A critical and chronological view of what has been published on the subject'.

AVOIDING BIASED COMPARISONS

To ensure that comparisons are fair, several sources of bias must be identified and minimised; if they are not, a new treatment might appear better than an existing one when in fact it is not.

In considering individual research studies, this could result from:

- comparing the progress of relatively well patients given a new treatment with the progress of relatively ill patients given a standard treatment
- biased assessment of the results of treatment – for example, by comparing the opinions of patients or doctors who know that they have used an expensive new treatment, and who think this is better, with the opinions of those who know that they have had an existing standard treatment

And in reviewing several similar studies, from:

- considering only studies that show a new treatment in a favourable light, without including other 'negative' studies that have either failed to confirm it has benefits, or suggest that it may be harmful ('negative' studies are often not reported)
- biased selection from and interpretation of the available evidence.

Often people trying to decide which treatments to use simply do not recognise that these biases result in unfair tests of treatments. Sadly, however, people with vested interests sometimes exploit biases to make treatments look as if they are better than they really are. This happens when some researchers – usually but not always for commercial reasons – deliberately ignore existing evidence. They design, analyse, and report studies to paint their own results for a particular treatment in a favourable light.

'Research sponsored by the drug industry was more likely to produce results favouring the product made by the company sponsoring the research than studies funded by other sources. The results apply across a wide range of disease states, drugs, and drug classes, over at least two decades and regardless of the type of research being assessed.'

Lexchin J, Bero LA, Djulbegovic B, Clark O. Pharmaceutical industry sponsorship and research outcome and quality: systematic review. *British Medical Journal* 2003;326:1167-70.

Biases due to differences in patients being compared

Comparisons of two treatments will be unfair if relatively well patients have received one of the treatments and relatively ill patients have received the other treatment. Occasionally this problem can be tackled by comparing different treatments given at different times to the same patient – a cross-over study. But there are many circumstances in which such studies are out of the question. For example, it is almost always impossible to compare different surgical operations in this way.

Treatments are usually tested by comparing groups of patients who have received different treatments. If these comparisons are to be fair, the groups of patients must be similar so that like will be compared with like. If those who receive a treatment are more likely to do well or badly than those receiving an alternative, this bias makes it impossible to be confident that any difference in results truly reflects an effect of the treatment rather than something that would have occurred anyway. The 18th-century surgeon William Cheselden was aware of this problem. In his day, surgeons were comparing death rates in their patients after operations to remove bladder stones. But Cheselden pointed out that older patients were more likely to die. So, to compare the frequency of deaths in groups of patients who had undergone various types of operation by different surgeons, it would be important to take account of any age differences among the patients on whom each surgeon had operated.

Comparing the experiences and outcomes of patients who happened to have received different treatments in the past is still used today as a way of trying to assess the effects of treatments. The challenge is to know whether the comparison groups were sufficiently alike before receiving treatment. For example, attempts to assess the effects of hormone replacement therapy (HRT) by comparing the frequencies of illnesses experienced by women using HRT with those in women not using it show how dangerously misleading this approach can be. Whereas these comparisons suggested that HRT reduced the risk of heart attacks and stroke, subsequent randomised trials showed that it had exactly the opposite effect (see Chapter 1). So research that had not taken account of these biases was not just useless, it harmed women too.

The best approach is to plan the comparisons before starting treatment. Before beginning his comparison of six treatments for scurvy on board HMS *Salisbury* in 1747, James Lind took care to select patients who were at a similar stage of this often lethal disease (see Chapter 1). He also ensured that they had the same basic diet and were accommodated in similar conditions. So, he clearly recognised that factors other than treatment might influence the sailors' chances of recovery.

Just as much care must be taken today to ensure that treatment comparison groups will be composed of similar people. And there is only one way to do this: some method based on chance must be used to assemble the groups. This 'random allocation' is the only but crucially important feature of the category of fair tests known as 'randomised' (see Chapter 4, box on page 59).

The techniques of drawing lots – for example, by using dice – will ensure that comparison groups are composed of patients who are similar, not just in terms of known and measured important factors such as age, but also of unmeasured factors that may influence recovery from illness, such as diet, occupation and other social factors, and anxiety about illness or proposed treatments. And the best way to avoid bias in allocating patients to comparison groups is to ensure that patients and their doctors do not know to which groups patients will be assigned.

After taking the trouble to assemble comparison groups in such a way that like will be compared with like, it is important to avoid introducing bias by ignoring the progress of some of the patients in these groups. This means that, as far as possible, all the patients allocated to the groups should be followed up and included in the main analysis of the results of the group

---

REASON TO RANDOMISE

'A doctor who contributes to randomised treatment trials should not be thought of as a research worker, but simply as a clinician with an ethical duty to his patients not to go on giving them treatments without doing everything possible to assess their true worth.'

Rees G, ed. *The friendly professional. Selected writings of Thurstan Brewin.*
Bognor Regis: Eurocommunica, 1996.

to which they were allocated – a so-called 'intention-to-treat' analysis – regardless of which treatment they actually received.

This approach may seem illogical, but ignoring it can make the tests unfair. Take the example of patients at risk of stroke owing to blockage of a blood vessel supplying the brain. Researchers conduct a test to find out whether an operation to unclog the blood vessel can reduce strokes in patients with dizzy spells as a result of the blockage – they compare people allocated to have the operation with those allocated not to have it. If they record the frequency of strokes only among patients who survive the immediate effects of the operation, the test will miss the important fact that the surgery itself can cause stroke and death. Consequently this will be an unfair test of the effects of the operation.

Biases in assessing treatment outcomes

Most patients and doctors hope that medical treatments will help. This optimism can have a very positive effect on everybody's satisfaction with medical care, as the British doctor Richard Asher noted in one of his essays for doctors:

> 'If you can believe fervently in your treatment, even though controlled tests show that it is quite useless, then your results are much better, your patients are much better, and your income is much better, too. I believe this accounts for the remarkable success of some of the less gifted, but more credulous members of our profession, and also for the violent dislike of statistics and controlled tests which fashionable and successful doctors are accustomed to display.'[46]

Even when doctors know that they are prescribing a treatment that has no 'physical' effects, they may do so in the hope that it will benefit their patients through psychologically mediated effects. In other words, patients who believe that a treatment will help to relieve their symptoms – even though the treatment is, in fact, a dummy drug (a placebo) – may well experience improvements in their condition.

So, when conducting fair tests of treatment, it is essential to reduce the biases that can occur when doctors and patients assess the results. The technique known as 'blinding' is commonly used to achieve this – and it has an interesting history. In the 18th century, Louis XVI of France called for an investigation into Anton Mesmer's claims about the beneficial effects of so-called animal magnetism (mesmerism). The king wanted to know whether the effects were due to any 'real' force or to 'illusions of the mind'. Blindfolded people were told either that they were or were not receiving mesmerism when in fact, at times, the reverse was happening.

The people who were tested only felt effects when they had been told that they were receiving the treatment.

For some outcomes – death, for example – biased assessment is very unlikely because there is little room for doubt about whether someone has died. However, the assessment of most outcomes either always, quite properly, involves subjectivity, as with patients' symptoms, or may involve it. For example, people may have individual reasons for preferring one of the treatments being compared over another: they may be more alert to signs of possible benefit when they believe a treatment is good for them, and more ready to ascribe harmful effects to a treatment about which they are worried.

In these common circumstances, blinding is desirable for fair tests. The two treatments being compared must therefore appear to be the same. Sometimes one of these is a placebo – a physically inactive (dummy) treatment. For instance, when the Medical Research Council first tested treatments for the common cold in the 1940s and 1950s, it would have been very difficult to interpret the results of the tests had identical-looking placebos not been used to prevent both patients and doctors knowing whether the patients were receiving the new drug or a placebo. This is known as a double-blind trial.

Double-blinding can be so important that it is worth considering another example. Researchers looked at the effects of blinding of doctors (keeping them unaware of whether patients were receiving the drug or a placebo) on the results of a clinical trial of treatments for multiple sclerosis. All the patients were examined by both a blinded and an unblinded doctor at each assessment during the trial; each doctor scored the results. The unblinded – but not the blinded – doctors' scores showed an apparent benefit for one of the treatments. However, use of the blinded doctors' scores prevented the wrong conclusions being drawn.[47] Overall, the greater the element of subjectivity in assessing outcomes, the greater is the need for blinding to make tests of treatments fair.

Sometimes, however, it is simply impossible to blind patients and doctors to the identity of the treatments being compared – for example, one can hardly disguise the difference between surgery and a drug treatment. Some unambiguous outcomes – death, for example – leave little scope for biased assessment. Even when bias might creep in – for example in assigning a cause of death – this can be done by people who do not know which treatments individual patients received.

HOW TO INTERPRET UNBIASED COMPARISONS

Taking account of differences between treatments intended and treatments received

For all the reasons given so far in this chapter, you will have realised by now that fair tests of treatments have to be planned carefully. The documents setting out these plans are known as protocols. Among other things, protocols specify details about the treatments to be compared. However, the best-laid plans may not work out quite as intended – the treatments actually received by patients sometimes differ from those that they should have received. For example, patients may not take treatments as intended; or one of the treatments may become unavailable. If such discrepancies are discovered, the implications need to be thought about and addressed carefully when the results are analysed and interpreted.

Taking account of the play of chance

When comparing two treatments, any differences in results may simply reflect the play of chance. Say five people improve with a new treatment and seven improve with the standard comparison treatment. No one could be confident that the new treatment was worse than the standard one. If the comparison was repeated, the numbers of patients who improve might be reversed (seven against five), or come out the same (six against six), or in some other ratio.

However, if 50 people improve with a new treatment and 70 improve with the standard treatment, chance becomes a less likely explanation for the difference. If 500 people improve with a new treatment and 700 improve with the standard treatment, clearly the new treatment is indeed worse than the standard one (and about half of new treatments are).

So, the way to make it less likely that people will be misled by the play of chance in treatment tests is to base conclusions on sufficiently large numbers of patients who either improve or deteriorate, or neither.

To assess the role that chance may have played in the outcomes of fair tests, researchers use 'tests of statistical significance'. These help to avoid drawing the mistaken conclusion that there are real differences in treatments when there are not and – a far more common danger – that there are no differences between treatments when there actually are. When researchers and statisticians talk about significant differences between treatments they are referring to statistical significance. But it is important to remember that statistical significance is not necessarily 'significant' in the usual sense of the word. A difference between treatments which is very unlikely to be due to chance – a statistically significant difference – may have no practical significance at all. For example, a systematic review of randomised studies comparing the experiences of tens of thousands of healthy men who took an aspirin a day with those of tens of thousands of other men who did not take aspirin found a lower rate of heart attacks among the aspirin takers. This difference was statistically significant, that is, it was unlikely to be explained by the play of chance. However, this finding is not necessarily of practical significance. If a healthy man's risk of having a heart attack is already very low, taking a drug in order to make it even lower may be unjustified, particularly as aspirin has side-effects.[48]

One approach to reducing the likelihood of being misled by the play of chance is to estimate something called confidence intervals. Confidence intervals give the range within which the true size of a treatment effect (which is never precisely known) lies, with a given degree of certainty (usually 95% or 99%). This is similar to asking the question 'How long does it take you to travel to work?' and getting the answer '20 minutes to an hour, depending on the traffic'.

So, statistical tests help to take account of the play of chance and avoid concluding that treatment differences exist when they do not or do not exist when they do.

DETECTING AND INVESTIGATING UNANTICIPATED EFFECTS OF TREATMENTS

Initial tests of treatments – for example, those required for licensing new drugs for public release – cover at most a few hundred or a few thousand people treated over a few months. Only relatively short-term and frequent unanticipated effects are likely to be picked up at this stage, whereas rare effects and those that take some time to develop will not be discovered until there has been more widespread use of treatments. When doctors prescribe a new drug more routinely, for example, their patients may differ from those who were selected to participate in the original tests: they may be older or younger, of a different sex, more or less ill, or suffering from other health problems in addition to the condition at which the treatment is targeted. Often unanticipated effects of treatments, whether bad or good, are first suspected by health professionals or patients. But which of these hunches reflect real effects?

If the unanticipated effect is very unusual and occurs quite often after the treatment has been used, it will generally strike both doctors and patients that something is wrong. This is what happened with thalidomide (see Chapter 1) – babies born without limbs were previously almost

If you have a bag (which you cannot see into) containing 30 sweets that could be either orange or white, then the number of orange sweets in the bag at the start could lie between nought and 30. The confidence interval (CI) for the number of orange sweets is 0-30.

If you drew a handful of sweets out of the bag and there are four orange and two white sweets in your hand then you know that there were at least four orange sweets at the start and no more than 28 – i.e., there were 30 sweets to begin with and you now know that at least two were white. So the CI for the number of orange sweets there were at the start is now 4-28.

If you grab another handful of sweets (without replacing the first handful) and pull out three orange and six white sweets, then the CI for the number of orange sweets in the bag at the start is 7-22. The next selection contains three orange and five white sweets, giving a CI of 10-17 for the number of orange sweets at the start. The selection after that contains just four orange sweets, giving a CI of 14-17. When the last three sweets are drawn out two are orange and one is white. So you can conclude that there were 16 orange sweets at the start. As the total number of sweets drawn out gets larger, so the CIs get shorter. This example calculates absolute CIs – at every stage one can be absolutely sure that the real number of orange sweets lies somewhere between the two confidence limits.

The diagram illustrates this example, showing how the CIs are narrowed at each step.

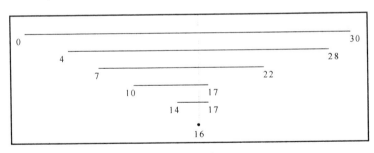

Adapted from Critical Appraisal Skills Programme, Cochrane Consumer (UK). Consumers commenting on Cochrane Reviews. Post-workshop pack. 2003-4, p23.

unheard of. Unanticipated beneficial effects are detected similarly – for example, when it was found that a drug used to treat schizophrenia also lowered cholesterol. When such striking relationships are noted, they will often be confirmed as real unanticipated effects of treatment.

However, most hunches about unanticipated effects of treatment are based on far less convincing evidence. As with studies designed to detect hoped-for effects of treatments, the planning of tests to confirm or dismiss less striking suspected unanticipated effects involves avoiding biased comparisons. Such tests must also observe the principle of comparing 'like with like'.

Sometimes researchers can conduct further analyses (or follow-up) of people who took part in earlier studies in which similar groups had been created by use of random allocation (see above). Usually this is not an option. So, assembling new unbiased comparison groups is more of a challenge. Here, the very fact that these effects were unanticipated actually helps pinpoint them. The unanticipated effect is usually a different condition or disease from the one for which the treatment was prescribed. For example, when hormone replacement therapy (HRT) was first introduced for relief of menopausal symptoms, a woman's risk of developing breast cancer was unlikely to have been taken into account. In other words, there was no obvious reason to expect that women who received HRT differed in their risk of developing breast cancer from those who did not. This was the basis for fair tests which showed that HRT increases the risk of breast cancer.[49]

When the suspected unanticipated effect relates to a treatment for a common condition such as heart attack but does not occur very often with the new treatment, the unanticipated effect will be found only by surveying large numbers of people receiving the treatment. For example, although some researchers thought that aspirin might reduce the risk of heart attack and began fair tests of their theory in patients in the late 1960s, most doctors thought that this was highly unlikely. They began to change their minds when a large study to detect unanticipated adverse effects of drugs showed that patients admitted to hospital with heart attacks were less likely than apparently similar patients to have recently taken aspirin.

The ground rules for detecting and investigating unanticipated effects of medical treatments were first set out clearly in the late 1970s in the wake of the thalidomide disaster. With many powerful treatments introduced since that time, this aspect of fair tests of medical treatments remains just as challenging and important today.

TAKING ACCOUNT OF ALL THE RELEVANT EVIDENCE

One of the pioneers of fair tests of treatments, the statistician Austin Bradford Hill, said that those reading research reports wanted answers to four questions:

- Why did you start?
- What did you do?
- What did you find?
- What does it mean anyway?

The answer to the last question is especially important since this is what influences actual choices and decisions about treatment and future research. A single fair test of treatment very seldom yields strong enough evidence to provide a confident answer. A fair test is usually only one of several addressing the same question. So, to answer 'what does it mean?', the evidence from one test must be interpreted alongside evidence from the other fair tests addressing the same or similar questions.

More than a century ago, the president of the British Association for the Advancement of Science, Lord Rayleigh, commented on the need to observe this principle:

> 'If, as is sometimes supposed, science consisted in nothing but the laborious accumulation of facts, it would soon come to a standstill, crushed, as it were, under its own weight . . . Two processes are thus at work side by side, the reception of new material and the digestion and assimilation of the old; and as both are essential we may spare ourselves the discussion of their relative importance. One remark, however, should be made. The work which deserves, but I am afraid does not always receive, the most credit is that in which discovery and explanation go hand in hand, in which not only are new facts presented, but their relation to old ones is pointed out.'[50]

Even today, however, Rayleigh's wise advice is routinely ignored. Consequently, it is often impossible for readers of new research reports to obtain a reliable answer to the question 'what does it mean?'. And reporting new test results without interpreting them in the light of other relevant evidence, reviewed systematically, can delay identification of both useful and harmful treatments. For example, between the 1960s and early 1990s, researchers carried out over 50 fair tests of drugs to reduce heart rhythm abnormalities in patients having heart attacks before it was realised that these drugs were killing people (see Chapter 1). Had each successive report assessed the new results in the context of all the other relevant evidence, the fatal effects of these drugs could have been identified a decade earlier.

Dealing with biased reporting of the available evidence

It is easy to state that the results of new research should be interpreted in the context of systematic reviews of all other relevant, reliable evidence, but this is a challenge in many ways – not least because some relevant evidence does not get published. Studies that have given 'disappointing' or 'negative' results are less likely to be reported than others. This 'reporting bias' stems principally from researchers not writing up or submitting reports of their research for publication. However, sometimes journals show bias when they reject submitted reports. There is an additional problem: researchers may selectively suppress those results that go against their interpretation of the treatment effects.

To reduce reporting biases, all fair tests of treatments need to be registered when they begin (see www.controlled-trials.com). Over and above this, all clinical trial results should be published – whether or not they are 'disappointing' to the sponsors of the research or the researchers themselves. Biased under-reporting of research is unscientific and un-ethical. Recent exposés of suppression of unwelcome evidence about the effects of drugs have led to major public scandals and court actions against pharmaceutical companies. These events have given force to long-standing demands that clinical trials be registered publicly at inception, and that all results be published. In the days before electronic publishing it was difficult to force compliance with these principles, but the advent of open-access electronic journals, such as those published by BioMed Central (www.biomedcentral.com) and the Public Library of Science (www. plos.org), has overcome this obstacle.

Avoiding biased selection from the available evidence

Biases can not only distort individual tests of treatments and lead to false conclusions but also distort reviews of evidence. Reviews are important because most people depend on them, but reviews must be done systematically otherwise they will be misleading. For example, reviewers could just draw on studies with which they were familiar; if they do, this is likely to bias their conclusions.

To avoid these problems, plans for systematic reviews should be set out in protocols, making clear what measures will be taken to reduce biases. These measures will include specifying: which questions about treatments the review will address; the criteria that will make a study eligible for inclusion in the review; the ways in which potentially eligible studies will be identified; and the steps that will be taken to minimise biases in selecting studies for inclusion in the review.

Systematic reviews addressing what appears to be the same question quite often reach different conclusions. Sometimes this is because the questions addressed are subtly different; sometimes it reflects differences in the methods used by the reviewers. In these circumstances it is important to judge which reviews are most likely to have reduced the effects of biases and the play of chance most successfully.

What if the reviewers have any other interests that might affect the conduct or interpretation of their review? Were they, for example, directly associated with the company that made the new drug being tested? When assessing the evidence for an effect of evening primrose oil on eczema, reviewers who were associated with the manufacturers reached far more enthusiastic conclusions than those with no such commercial interest (see Chapter 1).

Commercial interests are not alone in leading to biased selection from the available evidence for inclusion in reviews. We all have prejudices that can do this – researchers, health professionals, and patients alike.

Using meta-analysis to reduce the play of chance

To reduce the play of chance, the results from all the relevant studies can sometimes be combined statistically – this is known as a meta-analysis. Although methods for meta-analysis were developed by statisticians over many years, it was not until the 1970s that they began to be applied more extensively, initially by social scientists and then by medical researchers. By the end of the 20th century it had become widely accepted that meta-analysis was an important element of fair tests of treatments.

Meta-analysis is another way to help avoid erroneous conclusions that treatments have no effects when in fact they are either useful or harmful. Take the example of a short, inexpensive course of steroids given to women expected to give birth prematurely. The first randomised controlled trial – which showed a reduced likelihood of their babies dying – was reported in 1972. A decade later more trials had been done but these were small and the individual results were confusing, and, at that time, the evidence had not been combined in a systematic review using meta-analysis. If it had been, the result would have shown even stronger evidence favouring a beneficial effect of steroids. In fact, no systematic reviews using meta-analysis were published until 1989 – so most obstetricians had not realised the treatment was so effective and tens of thousands of premature babies had suffered and died unnecessarily.[51]

4

DEALING WITH UNCERTAINTY ABOUT THE EFFECTS OF TREATMENTS

Chapter 3 outlined how treatments should be tested fairly. In this chapter we take an in-depth look at the uncertainties that almost invariably surround treatment effects.

In the 1970s, one of the authors (IC), while holidaying in the USA, broke an ankle and was treated by an orthopaedic surgeon. The surgeon put the leg in a temporary splint, recommending that the next step, once the swelling had subsided, would be a lower leg plaster cast for six weeks. On returning home a couple of days later, IC went to the local fracture clinic, where a British orthopaedic surgeon, without hesitation, dismissed this advice. Putting the leg in plaster, the surgeon said, would be wholly inappropriate. In the light of this obvious uncertainty about which treatment was better, IC asked whether he could participate in a controlled comparison to find out. The British surgeon answered that controlled trials are for people who are uncertain whether or not they are right – and that he was certain.

How can such a pronounced difference in professional opinion come about, and what is a patient to make of this? Each surgeon was certain, individually, about the correct course of action. Yet their widely divergent views clearly revealed uncertainty within the profession as a whole about the best way to treat a common fracture. Was there good evidence about which treatment was better? If so, was one or neither surgeon aware of the evidence? Or was it that nobody knew which treatment was better? Perhaps the two surgeons differed in the value they placed on particular outcomes of treatments: the American surgeon may have been more concerned about relief of pain – hence the recommendation of a plaster cast – while his British counterpart may have been more worried about the possibility of muscle wasting, which occurs when a limb is immobilised in this way. If so, why did neither surgeon ask IC which outcome mattered more to him, the patient?

There are several separate issues here. First, was there any reliable evidence comparing the two very different approaches being recommended? If so, did it show their relative effects on outcomes (reduced pain, or reduced muscle wasting, for example) that might matter to IC or to other patients, who might have different preferences to his? But what if there was no evidence providing the information needed?

Some clinicians are clear about what to do when there is no reliable evidence. For example, one doctor who specialises in caring for people with stroke has put it this way: 'I can reassure a patient that I am an expert in stroke assessment and diagnosis, and that I can reliably interpret the brain scan, and order the correct tests. I also know from existing research that my patient will fare better if cared for in a stroke unit. However, there is one aspect of management that I and others are uncertain about, and that is whether I should be prescribing clot-busting drugs: these drugs may do more good than harm, but they may actually do more harm than good. In these circumstances I feel it is my duty to help reduce this uncertainty by explaining to my patient that I am only prepared to prescribe this treatment within the context of a carefully controlled comparison.'[52] In this chapter, we want to consider uncertainties of this kind – that is, when there is inadequate information about the effects of alternative treatments, and there are no strong patient preferences.

DRAMATIC EFFECTS: RARE AND READILY RECOGNISABLE

Uncertainties about the effects of treatments are almost inevitable – only rarely will the results be so dramatic that there is no room for doubt. When this does happen, the treatment effect is very obvious. This was the case when the sulphonamide group of antibiotics, discovered in the 1930s, were used to treat a then common cause of death in women during childbirth – 'childbed' or puerperal fever. Puerperal fever was caused by a bacterial infection of the genital tract, the usual culprit being the organism known as *Streptococcus pyogenes*. Despite the introduction of strict antiseptic practices in the late 1870s, puerperal fever still killed thousands of women worldwide. The use of sulphonamides had a dramatic effect – death rates plummeted. There was a similarly dramatic response when sulphonamides were used to treat the serious type of bacterial meningitis (inflammation of the membrane covering the brain) known as meningococcal meningitis – again, the plunging death rates left little room for doubt. In these cases, there was no need for carefully controlled tests to show the results of sulphonamide treatment – the effects were overwhelmingly obvious by comparison with the fate of patients in the pre-sulphonamide days.

Other dramatic effects include two that we mentioned in Chapter 3 – the use of opium to relieve pain, and insulin for diabetes. In the 1920s, for example, when the Canadian doctors Banting and Best discovered insulin (a hormone produced by the pancreas), patients with diabetes had short lives and suffered immensely, wasting away with uncontrollably high blood sugar levels. Very quickly, the initial results of animal tests led to the use of insulin in patients, with outstanding success – their response was near miraculous at the time.

Another example from that era was the use of liver – later shown to be a source of vitamin B12 – for patients with pernicious anaemia. In this then fatal type of anaemia, the red blood cells fall over time to disastrously low levels, leaving patients with a ghostly pallor and profound weakness. When these patients were given liver extract the results were rapid and effective, and now vitamin B12 is prescribed routinely. Similarly, in the 1940s, the beneficial effects of streptomycin for tuberculous meningitis and of penicillin for various bacterial infections were also unmistakable.

More recently, the effects of organ transplants in patients with kidney, liver, or heart failure, or hip replacements in patients with arthritic pain were so striking that carefully controlled tests were superfluous. And around the beginning of this century similarly dramatic results were seen in patients given imatinib for chronic myeloid leukaemia.[53] Before

'Early in 1943, at the British General Hospital in Bangalore, South India, we were instructed to make friendly contacts locally. The director of the city's Institute of Science and Technology took me on a tour that was indeed impressive. But what shook me was the encounter with two young biochemists who proudly displayed a flask of what looked like porridge that they claimed was penicillin: "we've read all the articles." Alongside was a dish with a heavy growth of streptococci, they said, and another quite clean whence they assured me that the same bacteria had been cleared by the "penicillin". In 1943 we knew a little about penicillin from the journals that arrived regularly from home and the USA and had the highest expectations of it.

Soon after we admitted an officer-cadet, in extremis, with infected cavernous sinus thrombosis and septicaemia [a widespread bacterial infection, also affecting blood vessels in the brain]. Our several surgeon-specialists would not touch him. We tried everything else to no avail.

It seemed a crazy idea, but what was the alternative? We discussed and discussed, doctors and nurses; there were no answers. Meanwhile the patient was increasingly comatose. We resolved to give him the chance.

So off on my bike to the Institute. I explained the situation and they readily gave me a flask of the gruel, a little thinned. We selected the widest bore needle in the hospital, filled a large syringe, and I somehow injected the stuff intramuscularly. Next morning the patient asked for tea. Recovery was uneventful. The one dose it appeared was enough.

Morris JN. Recalling the miracle that was penicillin: two memorable patients. *Journal of the Royal Society of Medicine* 2004;97:189-90.

imatinib was introduced, this type of leukaemia responded very poorly to standard treatments. When the new drug was tried in patients who had not responded to standard therapy, the results were dramatic.

MODERATE TREATMENT EFFECTS: USUAL AND NOT SO OBVIOUS

However, most treatments do not have dramatic effects and carefully controlled tests are needed to assess them. And sometimes a treatment may have a dramatic effect in some conditions but not in others. For example, whereas sulphonamides were hugely effective for the 'killer diseases' puerperal fever and meningococcal meningitis, their effects in disorders in which a substantial proportion of patients survived without the drugs were far more modest. To assess the results of sulphonamides in these cases it was necessary to use carefully controlled tests. Several clinical trials were done in the 1930s and 1940s showing that although sulphonamides had worthwhile effects in erysipelas (a severe bacterial skin infection) and pneumonia, they were unlikely to be useful in scarlet fever.[54]

Similarly, although vitamin B12 was undoubtedly effective for pernicious anaemia, dispute continues to this day about whether patients need monthly or quarterly injections. That question will only be answered by carefully controlled tests comparing the two options. And whereas the pain relief with hip replacements was dramatic, the relative merits of different types of artificial hip joints are far more subtle, but may nevertheless be important. For example, some may wear out faster than others.

WHEN PRACTITIONERS DISAGREE

Large variations in the therapies used for a given condition provide evidence for professional uncertainty about best treatment. Another example of uncertainty is the treatment of benign enlargement of the prostate gland. This condition – known as benign prostatic hyperplasia (BPH) – is common in older men. The most bothersome symptoms are frequency or difficulty in passing urine. There are several ways of treating BPH, including letting nature take its course – sometimes called 'watchful waiting' or 'active monitoring' – since the symptoms may improve spontaneously. Other non-surgical options include conventional drug treatment (several drugs are currently prescribed for BPH) and a natural plant product, *Serenoa repens*, which is an extract of the American saw palmetto or dwarf palm. Then there is surgery – and the rates of surgery for BPH vary considerably. In the USA, for example, when researchers collected evidence for operation rates by region of the country in 1996, they found that these ranged nearly fourfold – from six to 23 per thousand men enrolled in the largest American healthcare insurance scheme (Medicare).[55]

We know that the choice of treatments for BPH depends on preferences and trade-offs: individual men differ in their personal assessment of the risks and benefits. Those who choose surgery have the best chance of relieving their symptoms but face the risk of complications such as incontinence, retrograde (backwards) ejaculation, and impotence. Drug treatment is less successful at relieving symptoms but avoids the risks associated with surgery. And watchful waiting avoids the risks of surgery and drug treatment but is likely to leave symptoms unchanged. Controlled tests are needed to compare these options and thus help inform treatment decisions. When a man seeks advice for his troublesome symptoms, the pros and cons of each option need to be explained by his doctor so that they can agree on the most appropriate choice of treatment for him. It seems reasonable to assume that among regions of the USA there will be roughly the same proportion of men for whom the various options are most appropriate. Yet, as the widely divergent operation rates illustrate, doctors remain uncertain about whether, and if so when, to use surgery.

In prostate cancer too, as we described in Chapter 2, there is considerable uncertainty about the use of screening tests and, linked with that uncertainty, about treatment options.

Professional uncertainty also surfaces in the way in which tonsillectomy (surgical removal of the tonsils) is used for patients with chronic (persistent) tonsillitis or recurrent bouts of acute tonsillitis. In the past, tonsils were removed in children almost as a matter of routine, with scant regard paid to whether their symptoms, if any, merited surgery. Nowadays, tonsillectomy is used far more selectively but it is still a very common operation in children, and increasingly in adults. However, the indications for surgery are not generally agreed. Tonsillectomy is indicated for children whose breathing is severely affected by the enlarged tonsils. But in many countries numerous patients with recurrent acute tonsillitis, chronic tonsillitis, and recurrent non-specific 'sore throats' also have their tonsils removed. Although the presence of 'infection' is usually used to justify surgery, the frequency and severity of such infections vary considerably. And there are undoubtedly risks associated with surgery, over and above those generally associated with a general anaesthetic, including severe bleeding. Faced with these obvious variations in the use of tonsillectomy, a

Sir,

The one thing that is certain about the screening, diagnosis and treatment of prostate cancer is the uncertainty attached to it. It is life-threatening for some men and not for many others. So, whilst potentially 'curable' it may not need to be.

Recent correspondence reveals how difficult it is for men when they try to reconcile decisions with the evidence and opinions of scientific and medical experts. Hundreds of men are trying to do this every week. One man, Jeremy Laurance, says he'll hang on to his prostate for the moment, though he does seem to be ignoring symptoms to defy a cancer diagnosis when a trip to the GP is much more likely to confirm a benign and treatable prostate problem than it is to reveal cancer. Professor Robert Eisenthal feels grateful that he has had his removed. And, barring perhaps Jeremy's lack of interest in help from his GP, there are not many urologists or oncologists who'd state that either a man is obviously right or obviously wrong. Until unequivocal medical scientific evidence emerges this really is the best that these men and the others faced with these dilemmas each week, can do.

The key is the informed man or the best approximation of him possible. The only way to reduce the uncertainty is long-term support of research. In the mean time, we need broader policy to support men's health, which is not a specific government target at the moment, to help men engage with their own wellbeing and learn to be 'health literate' in the vernacular of the recent Wanless paper on public health.

Dr Chris Hiley, Head of Policy and Research, The Prostate Cancer Charity
Hiley C. Prostate dilemma [Letter]. *The Independent*, 2004, Jun 7, p26.

group of researchers decided to review, systematically, the controlled trials that had been done to address the uncertainty. They found that no clinical trials of tonsillectomy in adults had ever been done. The situation with respect to children was not much better: the researchers identified two studies but each had limitations. In one study, for example, children in the surgery groups – tonsillectomy alone or with removal of the adenoids (adenoidectomy) as well – differed from those who did not have surgery: the surgical groups had a different pattern of preceding throat infection and also came from poorer families. Clearly like was not being compared with like. The researchers therefore concluded that the effectiveness of tonsillectomy had not been adequately evaluated and that further controlled trials were needed.[56]

Once again, the treatment of breast cancer (see Chapter 2) provides an outstanding example of professional uncertainty. Although there has been much research into breast cancer diagnosis and therapy over the years, the wide variations in the interpretation of screening mammograms and in the use of surgery, radiotherapy, and chemotherapy indicate that many uncertainties remain. There are numerous unanswered questions about the basic biological features of the disease such as the role of genes, enzymes, or differences in patients' metabolism. The best treatment of very early stage breast cancers and 'pre-breast cancers' is unresolved, as is the ideal number of lymph nodes to remove from the armpit. Optimum organisation of screening and treatment services remains contentious, and so requires more evidence to inform practice. And as if that long list were not enough, topics of particular interest to patients, such as relief of fatigue associated with therapy, or the best way of treating lymphoedema – a distressing and disabling aftermath of surgery and radiotherapy in the armpit – still have not been tested adequately.

So where do we go from here? First, doctors need to weigh the best available evidence about a treatment from collective experience and systematic reviews of any reliable research studies that exist. Then they must discuss the options with their patients and be as clear as possible about the patients' preferences. If uncertainty remains after doing this, they need to acknowledge it and be prepared to explain to their patients why this is so. Rather than uncertainty being an admission of 'defeat' it should be seized upon as a prerequisite for progress, with the aim of making treatments more appropriate and safer. Then patients and clinicians must work together to design better research (see Chapter 7). Meanwhile patients need to understand that if, having looked at the evidence, their doctor says 'I

In 2002, a 58-year-old woman from New Jersey, USA, commented:

'Sadly, in my experience anyway, I have found it impossible to have a rational conversation with a physician, where my concerns are respected on the topic of mammograms, as the *New York Times* article says a patient should have. Doctors get belligerent and almost hostile if I say I have reservations about getting a yearly mammogram. The upshot is that I don't feel I have a good relationship with a physician, and that is not good. A good scientist is not afraid to express uncertainty on a topic or to discuss a topic openly. I'm afraid the practising physicians who I have come across do not have that scientific mindset.

Diane Palacios in correspondence with Dr D A Berry of the MD Anderson Cancer Center, University of Texas, 2002 (reproduced with permission).

Ms Palacios also wrote a letter directly to the *New York Times*, concluding 'I can live with uncertainty. I do not wish to live with dishonesty'.

Palacios D. Re: Senators hear from experts, then support mammography (news article March 1). *New York Times*, 2002 Mar 4, pA20.

Writing in 2005, a British junior doctor who had lately become a patient herself noted:

'Having worked in the NHS I had realistic expectations with regard to waiting, the uncertainties of diagnosis, and the time pressures on doctors. What I valued above all was being diagnosed and treated by individuals I could trust – by doctors who laid out the facts and uncertainties as known, told me the plan for the next stage and did not dress it up in a fancy box tied with a bow or distract me with talk of possible things that could go wrong or continuously ask me how I was feeling . . . "I am lucky", I told my father (a paediatrician); but he pointed out that I was not lucky – my experience should be the norm.'

Chambers C. Book review. Hippocratic oaths – medicine and its discontents. *Journal of the Royal Society of Medicine* 2005; 98: 39-40.

don't know', this is not the signal to seek a second opinion from another doctor who confidently says 'I do know' while blatantly ignoring the prevailing uncertainty.

So how should we cope with important uncertainty about the effects of a new drug or technique? An obvious answer is to try to reduce the uncertainty – by using the new form of care only within the context of research that has been designed to find out more about its effects. A medical ethicist put it this way:

> 'If we are uncertain about the relative intrinsic merits of any [different] treatments, then we cannot be certain about those merits in any given use of one of them – as in treating an individual patient. So it seems irrational and unethical to insist one way or another before completion of a suitable trial. Thus the answer to the question, "What is the best treatment for the patient?" is: "The trial". The trial is the treatment. Is this experimentation? Yes. But all we mean by that is choice under uncertainty, plus data collection. Does it matter that the choice is "random"? Logically, no. After all, what better mechanism is there for choice under uncertainty?'[57]

If no such trial is available, at the very least the results of using new and untested treatments should be recorded in a standardised way so that they can contribute to the body of knowledge for the benefit of the patients receiving the untested treatment and patients everywhere. Since billions of pounds of taxpayers' money have been invested in NHS information systems, it is not unreasonable to expect them to be used for the benefit of the public in this way.

There are several examples of health professionals using this responsible approach. In the 1980s, British and Canadian obstetricians agreed that they would only use chorionic villus sampling – an invasive new technique for antenatal diagnosis of fetal abnormalities – within controlled trials until more was known about its safety compared with alternatives, such as amniocentesis (see Chapter 7). Similarly, in the 1990s, British paediatricians agreed that babies born with oxygen starvation should be treated with new heart-lung machines only within a randomised controlled trial. By doing this, doctors and parents would find out promptly whether the new machines were better or worse than the current best standard care in reducing the likelihood of infant death or severe disability. More recently, paediatricians have applied the same approach to assess suggestions that cooling ill newborn babies may help to protect them from brain damage. These disciplined approaches by doctors reflect their recognition that, when there is uncertainty about treatment effects, it is all too easy to do unintended harm while acting with the best of intentions.

Although there is now increasing interest in promoting this attitude, particularly for new and often very expensive treatments, sadly, opportunities continue to be missed. For example, there is currently no known effective treatment for the devastating and rapidly fatal nervous system condition known as Creutzfeldt-Jakob disease (CJD), one form of which probably results from eating beef from cattle with mad cow disease (BSE). Understandably, relatives of people struck down with the condition

'Only because we do not know what the future holds can we have our hope and choices. In the context of informing patients about the effects of treatments, this means that the patients' basic right is whether to accept that uncertainty exists (which in practice often means disagreement among their doctors), and the proposed method for resolution of the existing uncertainties (which can include enrolment into a clinical trial as one means to resolve uncertainties).

Therefore uncertainty should not be looked on as the enemy but rather as a friend (or as the opportunity). Once uncertainty is recognised and acknowledged, more effective solutions for its resolution can be devised. Hence, "two cheers for uncertainty".'

Djulbegovic B. Paradox exists in dealing with uncertainty.
British Medical Journal 2004;328:1018.

sometimes call for any treatment to be tried that may hold out hope, even when little or nothing is known about the balance between possible success and possible harms (see Chapter 7). Yet how much more could be learnt, for patients' benefit, if such treatments were properly evaluated by fair tests.

REDUCING UNCERTAINTIES ABOUT THE EFFECTS OF TREATMENTS

There will have to be changes if uncertainties about the effects of treatments are to be reduced more effectively and efficiently. We discuss some of these – particularly the greater involvement of patients – in the last two chapters of the book. However, there is a particular issue – we touched on it above – that we want to raise here. When there is insufficient information about the effects of a treatment, knowledge can be increased by ensuring that doctors only offer it within the context of a formal evaluation until more is known about its value and possible disadvantages. So why do some prevailing attitudes actually discourage this risk-limiting approach?

The problem vexed a British paediatrician over 30 years ago when he pithily observed that he needed permission to give a treatment to half his patients (that is, to find out about its effects by giving half the patients the new treatment and half the existing treatment in a controlled comparison), but not if he wanted to give the treatment to all of them as a standard prescription.[58] This illogical double standard still pops up repeatedly and discourages clinicians who want to reduce uncertainties about the effects of treatments. For example, referring to treatments offered in routine practice, the General Medical Council (GMC) advises doctors: 'the amount of information you give each patient will vary, according to factors such as the nature of the condition, the complexity of the treatment, the risks associated with the treatment or procedure and the patient's own wishes.'[59] This flexibility is noticeably lacking in the GMC's guidance on consent to research, which states that people being invited to participate in clinical trials must be given 'the fullest possible information'.

It is important – and ethical – to consider the interests of *everyone* currently receiving treatment, not just the few who participate in controlled trials.[60] Clearly all relevant information should be available on request, but it is also desirable to tailor provision to a patient's individual preferences and requirements, which may change over time. Dogmatic insistence on full information and consent in all circumstances could well interfere with common sense and good practice.[61]

Patients requiring treatment and care, whether in clinical trials or not, are presumably equally variable in the amount of information they desire and their ability to understand it in the time available, and in their degree of anxiety and fear. When clinicians endeavouring to reduce uncertainties about the effects of treatments are forced to give 'the fullest possible information', they may severely upset those patients who prefer to 'leave it to the doctor'.[62] Investment in improving the communication skills of health professionals would be a better strategy than rigid insistence on full disclosure. Much more useful would be a flexible approach which recognises that trust between doctor and patient is the bedrock of any satisfactory consultation. The GMC (see above), which is currently revising its guidance on consent, would do better to recommend that people being invited to join a clinical trial be given *every opportunity of easy access to* the fullest possible information.

If a clinician tries a new therapy with the idea of studying it carefully, evaluating outcomes, and publishing the results, he or she is doing research. The subjects [sic] of such research are thought to be in need of special protection. The protocol must be reviewed by an Institutional Review Board (IRB) [equivalent to a research ethics committee in the UK]. The informed consent form will be carefully scrutinised and the research may be forbidden. On the other hand, a clinician may try this new therapy without any intention of studying it, merely because he believes it will be of benefit to his patients. In that situation, trying the new therapy is not research, the trial does not need IRB approval, and consent may be obtained in a manner governed only by the risk of malpractice litigation.

It would seem that the patients in the second situation (nonresearch) are at much higher risk than are the patients in the first situation (being part of formal clinical research). Furthermore, the physician in the first situation seems more ethically admirable. The physician in the first situation is evaluating the therapy, whereas the physician in the second situation is using the therapy based on his or her imperfect hunches. Nevertheless, because ethical codes that seek to protect patients focus on the goal of creating generalizable knowledge, they regulate the responsible investigator but not the irresponsible adventurer.

Lantos J. Ethical issues – how can we distinguish clinical research from innovative therapy? *American Journal of Pediatric Hematology/Oncology* 1994;16:72-5.

Being able to explain uncertainty clearly demands skills and a certain degree of humility on the part of doctors. Many feel uneasy when trying to explain to potential participants in a clinical trial that no one knows which treatment is best.[63, 64] But the public's attitude has changed: arrogant doctors who 'play God' are increasingly given short shrift. We need to focus on training doctors who are not ashamed to admit they are human and that they need the help and the participation of patients in research to provide more certainty about choices of treatments.

The main stumbling block for many health professionals and patients is lack of understanding about randomisation – why it is necessary, and what it means in practical terms (see Chapter 3). This highlights the urgency for accessible, clearly written information about clinical trials and why they are needed.

There are two distinct needs: first, general education to improve understanding about randomised controlled trials, and why they are

'Good morning Mrs Jones, my name is Dr Smith. Please sit down and make yourself comfortable. Your general practitioner has probably explained to you that he has asked me to see you because your breathlessness doesn't seem to be getting any better, and he wondered whether I might be able to suggest ways of helping. I hope I will be able to do so, but this may well mean seeing you on a number of occasions over the next few months and working together to find the best treatment for your condition.

I'm more likely to be able to help if I can get to know more about you and your priorities and preferences. As this is the first time we've met, I thought it might be helpful to mention briefly how I will try to do this. Patients vary in the amount of information that they want to give to and receive from their doctors. Most patients seem to get less information from their doctors than they want; but there are others who would rather not be told some of the things that some doctors assume that they must want to know. Because you and I don't know each other yet, I'm going to need your help in learning how much information you want about your problem, and about the possible treatment options. I'm going to depend on you to prompt me to give you more information if you think I'm not being sufficiently forthcoming, or to tell me that you've heard enough if you think I'm overdoing it. You also need to know that I will never lie in response to a straight question from you, and if I don't know the answer I will do my best to find it for you. Does that seem to you to be an acceptable way of proceeding?'

Oxman AD, Chalmers I, Sackett DL. A practical guide to informed consent to treatment.
British Medical Journal 2001;323:1464-6.

done; second, information about the reason for offering a patient treatment within a specific clinical trial. In waiting areas in clinics, people should be able to pick up simple leaflets about the need for clinical trials.[65] These could help to sow the seeds of understanding, and lessen the shock of an invitation to join a trial. Above all, controlled trials should be promoted as a partnership between health professionals and patients in order to improve treatment choices and quality of life. Then patients invited to participate in a trial should be told what this will involve, and why they are eligible. We would like to see the day when patients are not surprised to receive such an invitation: rather they would automatically ask which trials they might be eligible for,[66] and to judge whether the research questions are important for them.

'Randomisation is to minimise bias and ensure that the patients in each treatment group are as similar as possible in all known and unknown factors. This will ensure that any differences found between the groups in the outcome(s) of interest are due to differences in treatment effect and not differences between the patients receiving each of the treatments.

It removes the chance that a clinician will consciously or unconsciously allocate one treatment to a particular type of patient and the other treatment to another type, or that a certain kind of patient will choose one treatment whilst another kind will choose the other.

Harrison J. Presentation to Consumers' Advisory Group for Clinical Trials, 1995.

ETHICS, RESEARCH ETHICS COMMITTEES, AND THE INTERESTS OF PATIENTS

Strange as it may seem, medical ethicists and research ethics committees have helped to sustain the double standard on consent when there is uncertainty about the effects of treatments.[67] Ethicists often seem more concerned with protecting 'the vulnerable' than with encouraging the proper contribution of patients through equal partnerships. But as one medical ethicist has noted, 'If ethicists and others want something to criticise in clinical trials, they should look at scientifically inadequate work, reinvention of wheels, and above all, unjustifiable exclusions and unjust and irrational uses of resources. The present debate is flawed by a failure to take note of what trials are for – to make sure that the treatments we use are safe, and do what they do better than the alternatives. There are no short cuts in ethics – no more than in trials.'[68]

Research ethics committees – independent committees that evaluate ethical aspects of proposals for new research – evolved in response to various scandals of clearly unethical experiments on people, from the 1930s onwards. These committees have been very important in protecting people from abuses perpetrated in the name of research, and also in scrutinising the type of research designed to increase scientific knowledge, but not primarily to assess the effectiveness of treatments. However, when it comes to treatments offered in the context of controlled trials, they are serving patients poorly:[69]

Now that an international meta-register of controlled trials has been established (www.controlled-trials.com, accessed, Aug 9, 2000), the framework exists for creating a consumer-led, electronic *Good Controlled Trials Guide*, to help people who are considering participating in trials to make well-informed choices. Consumer commentaries on trials in the register could cover, for example, the importance of the questions being addressed, whether these had already been answered satisfactorily by previous research, whether the design of the study was scientifically and ethically robust, whether the primary outcomes chosen mattered to patients, and whether arrangements were in place for communicating the results of the research to those who had participated in it. Mobilization of consumer influence in this way might help to reorientate the clinical research agenda to serve the interests of patients better, just as Sheila Kitzinger's *Good Birth Guide*, for example, helped to make British maternity hospitals more aware of the public image of the care each of them was providing.

Chalmers I. A patient-led *Good Controlled Trials Guide, Lancet* 2000;356:774.

- They have not distinguished sufficiently between research assessing the effects of treatments that have hardly been used at all (indeed, which may not even have been licensed) and those that are already in widespread use;
- They have done little or nothing to draw attention to the double standard on consent to treatment which we have discussed above;
- They have not ensured that new research proposals are informed by systematic reviews of existing research;
- They have not required researchers to declare conflicts of interests; and
- They have done nothing to reduce biased under-reporting of research results.

So, there are serious questions about the extent to which research ethics committees are serving the best interests of the public. National Health Service governance arrangements go some way towards ensuring that the full results of approved studies are publicly available. For example, every research ethics committee should now keep a register of all proposals that it reviews and should request a final report from the researchers, to be delivered within three months. But there are still many shortcomings that

'From an ethical standpoint, clinical research and clinical practice should be considered congruent. This is so for very new forms of care intended to benefit patients (but whose potential for benefit or harm is unknown), as well as for more established forms of care, with which experience may be greater, but which are of unproven value. For the NHS, the ethical imperative is to encourage the research necessary to know how to use its limited resources to the best advantage of all in its care.'

Advisory Group on Health Technology Assessment. Assessing the Effects of Health Technologies: Principles, Practice, Proposals. London: Department of Health, 1992, p25.

need to be addressed to ensure that the work of research ethics committees is adequate and transparent. Only then will patients who are invited to participate in research on the effects of treatments have confidence that the studies are worthwhile, and that their contributions will be useful.

KEY POINTS
- Uncertainties about the effects of treatment are very common
- When we find that nobody knows the answer to an important uncertainty about the effects of treatment, we need to take steps to reduce the uncertainty
- Careful recording and evaluation, and well-conducted clinical trials are essential
- Double standards on consent to treatment within and outside clinical trials do not serve the interests of patients
- Much more could be done to help patients contribute to reducing uncertainties about the effects of treatments
- Research ethics committees are not currently serving the interests of patients effectively

5

CLINICAL RESEARCH: THE GOOD, THE BAD, AND THE UNNECESSARY

In earlier chapters we emphasised why research must be designed properly and address questions that matter to patients and the public. When it does, everyone can take pride and satisfaction in the results, even when hoped-for benefits do not materialise, because important insights will have been gained and uncertainty lessened. Much clinical research is good – and it is getting steadily better as it conforms with design and reporting standards. Nevertheless, bad and unnecessary research continues to be done and published for various reasons.

GOOD RESEARCH

Stroke is a leading cause of death and long-term disability. The death rate is between one in six and two in six during a first stroke, rising to four in six for subsequent strokes, most of which occur within a year of a first attack and affect the same region of the brain. One of the underlying causes of stroke is narrowing (stenosis) of the carotid artery that provides blood to the brain. The fatty material that coats the inside of the carotid artery sometimes breaks away, blocking smaller arterial tributaries, and thus causing a stroke. In the 1950s surgeons began to use an operation known as carotid endarterectomy to remove these fatty deposits. The hope was that surgery would reduce the risk of stroke. As with any operation, however, there is a risk of complications from the surgical procedure itself.

Although carotid endarterectomy became increasingly popular, it was not until the 1980s that randomised controlled trials were set up to assess the risks and benefits of surgery. Clearly this knowledge would be vitally important for patients and their doctors. Two well-designed trials – one in Europe and the other in North America – were carried out in patients who already had symptoms of carotid artery narrowing (minor stroke or fleeting stroke-like symptoms) to compare surgery with the best available non-surgical treatment. Several thousand patients took part in these long-term studies. The results, published in the 1990s, showed that surgery can reduce the risk of stroke or death but that benefit depends on the degree of narrowing of the carotid artery. Patients with relatively minor narrowing were, on balance, harmed by surgery, which can itself cause stroke. These important findings had direct implications for clinical practice.[70, 71]

Another outstanding example of good research concerns pregnant women. Worldwide, about 600,000 women die each year of pregnancy-related complications. Most of these deaths occur in developing countries and many are linked to pregnancy-associated convulsions (fits), a condition known as eclampsia. Eclampsia is a devastating illness that can kill both mother and baby. Women with the predisposing condition – pre-eclampsia (also known as toxaemia) – have high blood pressure and protein in their urine.

In 1995, research showed that injections of magnesium sulphate, a simple and cheap drug, could prevent recurrent fits in women with eclampsia (see Chapter 6). The same trial also showed that magnesium sulphate was better than other standard anticonvulsant drugs in stopping convulsions. So, the researchers knew it was important to find out whether magnesium sulphate could prevent convulsions in women with pre-eclampsia. The Magpie trial, designed to answer this question, was a major achievement, involving more than 10,000 pregnant women with pre-eclampsia in 33 countries around the globe. In addition to normal medical care, half the women received an injection of magnesium sulphate and half a placebo (dummy drug). Magpie gave clear and convincing results. It showed that magnesium sulphate more than halved the risk of convulsions. In addition, although the treatment did not apparently reduce the baby's risk of death, there was evidence that it could reduce the risk of the mother dying. And apart from minor side-effects, magnesium sulphate did not appear to harm the mother or the baby.[72, 73]

The results of good research are also making a real difference to the lives of children infected with HIV (human immunodeficiency virus), the cause of AIDS. Over 1,000 children die every day from HIV and AIDS-related illnesses across the world. Bacterial infections, such as pneumonia, which are associated with the children's weakened immune system, are a common cause of death. Co-trimoxazole is a widely available, low-cost antibiotic that has been used for many years to treat children and adults with chest infections unrelated to AIDS. Studies in adults with HIV also showed that the drug reduces other complications from bacterial infections.[74]

When preliminary evidence showed that the infections in children with HIV might also be reduced, a group of British researchers got together with colleagues in Zambia to test the effectiveness of co-trimoxazole as a preventive medicine in a large study in that country. The trial, which started in 2001 and lasted about two years, compared the antibiotic with a placebo in over 500 children. The results became clear sooner than anticipated when it was shown that the drug cut AIDS-related deaths by 43% and reduced the need for hospital admissions by 23%. At this point the independent committee scrutinising the results recommended that the trial be stopped. One immediate outcome was that all children in the trial were given co-trimoxazole as part of a Zambian government initiative. A wider consequence was that the World Health Organisation and UNICEF promptly altered their advice on effective medicines for children with HIV.[75, 76]

BAD RESEARCH

Regrettably, research is not always well done or relevant. Take the example of a distressing condition known as tardive dyskinesia. This is a serious side-effect associated with long-term use of drugs called neuroleptics (antipsychotics) which are prescribed for psychiatric disorders, and especially schizophrenia. The most prominent features of tardive dyskinesia are repetitive, involuntary movements of the mouth and face –

grimacing, lip smacking, frequent poking out of the tongue, and puckering or blowing out of the cheeks. Sometimes this is accompanied by twitching of the hands and feet. One in five patients taking a neuroleptic for more than three months experiences these side-effects.

In the 1990s a group of researchers began exploring, systematically, what treatments had been used for tardive dyskinesia over the preceding 30 years. Writing in 1996, they were rather surprised to have identified about 500 randomised controlled trials involving 90 different drug treatments. Yet none of these trials had produced any useful data. Some of the trials had included too few patients to give any reliable results; in others the treatments had been given so briefly as to be meaningless.[77]

The same research group went on to publish a comprehensive survey of the content and quality of controlled trials relevant to the treatment of schizophrenia in general. They looked at 2,000 trials and were disappointed in what they found. Over the years, drugs have certainly improved the prospects for people with schizophrenia in some respects. For example, most patients can now live at home or in the community. Yet, even in the 1990s (and still today), most drug trials were done on patients in hospital, so their relevance to outpatient treatment is uncertain. On top of that, the inconsistent way in which outcomes of treatment were assessed was astonishing. The researchers discovered that over 600 treatments – mainly drugs but also psychotherapy, for example – were tested in the trials, yet 640 different scales were used to rate the results and 369 of these were used only once. Comparing outcomes of different trials was therefore severely hampered and the results were virtually uninterpretable by doctors or patients. Among a catalogue of other problems, the researchers identified many studies that were too small or short term to give useful results. And new drug treatments were often compared with a drug well known for its side-effects – an obviously unfair test. The authors of this review concluded that half a century of studies of limited quality, duration, and clinical utility left much scope for well-planned, properly conducted, and competently reported trials.[78]

BEING BETTER INFORMED

'Even if evidence for the efficacy of interventions is lacking, or of poor quality, it is important to avoid nihilism. By undertaking systematic reviews and highlighting what high quality evidence does – or does not – exist, clinicians, researchers, policy-makers and patients will, at least, be better informed.'

Soares K, McGrath J, Adams C. Evidence and tardive dyskinesia.
Lancet 1996;347;1696-7.

The importance of assessing outcomes that matter to patients is clearly illustrated – in a very negative fashion – by early trials of epidural analgesia given to women for pain relief during labour. In the 1990s researchers reviewed the experience with controlled trials of epidural versus non-epidural analgesia. They estimated that, despite millions of women having been offered an epidural block over the preceding 20 years, fewer than 600 appeared to have participated in reasonably unbiased comparisons with other forms of pain relief. They identified nine comparison trials that could be confidently analysed. The comparisons were commonly measured in terms of levels of hormones and other substances believed to reflect stress during labour. Outcomes for the baby were also the focus of some attention. Yet any comparison of the pain reported by the women themselves was absent in all but two of the trials. In other words, those conducting the trials had largely overlooked an outcome that was surely of supreme importance – whether the women's pain was relieved or not.[79]

In Chapter 3 we explained how selective reporting of the results of research can lead to serious biases. Some 'negative' studies are totally suppressed when the results do not match the expectations of the investigators or funders. Without a published report to tell the tale, these trials disappear without trace. Another problem concerns selective reporting of results within published trials – that is, some of the results are excluded because they do not support the trialists' or funders' interpretation of the effects of the treatments being tested. This is indefensible. But why is biased under-reporting of research so important?

In 2004, a group of researchers reported the first thorough evaluation of this type of reporting bias.[80] They looked at over 100 randomised trials for which they could obtain copies of the trial plans, known as protocols, and any protocol amendments. So, they knew what outcomes the trialists had planned to assess. Then they looked at the published reports of these same trials and were taken aback at what they discovered. They found incomplete reporting of half of the outcomes relating to the beneficial effects of treatments and two thirds of those relating to harmful treatment effects.

They followed up this research by sending questionnaires to the trialists inquiring about the unreported outcomes. Fewer than half the trialists replied. Of these, the vast majority initially denied the existence of the missing outcomes even though there was incontrovertible evidence that they had existed at the outset of the research – they had been mentioned in the protocols and sometimes even in the methods sections of the published articles. To stamp out this bad practice the researchers called for the registration of all planned trials and for trial protocols to be publicly available for scrutiny.

'Outcome reporting bias acts in addition to the selective publication of entire studies and has widespread implications. It increases the prevalence [frequency] of spurious results, and reviews of the literature will therefore tend to overestimate the effects of interventions. The worst possible situation for patients, healthcare professionals, and policy-makers occurs when ineffective or harmful interventions are promoted, but it is also a problem when expensive therapies, which are thought to be better than cheaper alternatives, are not truly superior.'

Chan A-W, Hróbjartsson A, Haahr MT, Gøtzsche PC, Altman DG.
Empirical evidence for selective reporting of outcomes in randomized trials:
comparison of protocols to published articles.
Journal of the American Medical Association 2005;291:2457-65.

UNNECESSARY RESEARCH

Some research falls in between good and bad – it is plainly unnecessary. An example of such research concerns premature babies. When babies are born prematurely their lungs may be underdeveloped, with the risk of life-threatening complications such as respiratory distress syndrome. By the early 1980s there was overwhelming evidence that giving a steroid drug to pregnant women at risk of giving birth prematurely reduced the frequency of respiratory distress syndrome and death in newborn babies. Yet over the ensuing decade trials continued to be done in which steroids were compared with a placebo or no treatment. If the results of earlier trials had been reviewed systematically and combined by the technique of meta-analysis (see Chapter 3), it is unlikely that many of the later trials would have been started – the collective evidence would have shown that there was simply no need.

We mentioned another example of unnecessary research in Chapter 1, yet again because the results of preceding studies had not been gathered together and analysed. The treatment was the drug nimodipine, which was tested in stroke patients to reduce the extent of brain damage. In this example, the results of animal experiments had never been reviewed systematically and scrutinised properly. When they were, problems such as lack of randomisation and unblinded assessment of outcomes were obvious. The 'encouraging' results reported in animals that had led to the studies in stroke patients were found to be severely wanting.[81]

Yet another example of unnecessary research concerns patients undergoing bowel surgery. In 1969, a trial was done to see whether antibiotics – compared with placebos (dummy drugs) – reduced the risk of death after the operation. This was a small study and the results were inconclusive. Quite properly, further trials were done in the 1970s to reduce this uncertainty. As the evidence mounted, it became clear by the mid-1970s that antibiotics did indeed reduce the risk of death after surgery. Even so, trials continued to be approved by ethics committees and done by researchers throughout the 1980s to address the very same question. As a result, half the patients in these later studies were denied a treatment that had been shown to reduce their risk of dying after operations. How could this have happened? The most likely explanation is that trialists embarking on the later studies did not review the accumulated evidence systematically, or present the results of new research in the context of an up-to-date review of all the relevant evidence. Clearly, research ethics committees had not required researchers to have done so before approving the new studies. In other words, neither researchers nor ethics committees had put the interests of patients first.[82]

KEY POINTS

- Unnecessary research is a waste of time, effort, money, and other resources
- New research should only proceed if an up-to-date review of preceding research suggests that it is necessary
- Evidence from new research should be used to update a review of all the relevant results

6

LESS RESEARCH, BETTER RESEARCH, AND RESEARCH FOR THE RIGHT REASONS

An editorial in the *British Medical Journal* some years ago carried an arresting title: 'The scandal of poor medical research'.[83] The author called for less research, better research, and research done for the right reasons. In earlier chapters we have shown the kind of things that were bothering him.

LESS RESEARCH

For most of the organisations supporting biomedical research and most of the researchers doing it, their stated aim is straightforward: to contribute information to improve people's health. But how many of the millions of biomedical research reports published every year really do make a useful contribution to this worthy cause?

Researchers in Bristol decided to pose a fundamental question: 'To what extent are questions of importance to patients with osteoarthritis of

---

A MOUNTAIN OF INFORMATION

'Over two million articles are published annually in the biomedical literature in over 20,000 journals – literally a small mountain of information . . . In a stack, [the articles] would rise 500 metres.'

Mulrow CD. Rationale for systematic reviews.
In: Chalmers I, Altman CD, eds. *Systematic reviews*. London: BMJ Books, 1995.

---

the knee and the clinicians looking after them reflected in the research on this condition?'[84] They began by convening four focus groups – of patients, rheumatologists, physiotherapists, and general practitioners, respectively. These groups were unanimous in making clear that they did not want any more trials sponsored by pharmaceutical companies comparing yet another non-steroidal anti-inflammatory drug (the group of drugs that includes, for example, ibuprofen) against a placebo (dummy drug). Instead of drug trials, participants in the focus groups wanted rigorous evaluation of physiotherapy and surgery, and assessment of the educational and coping strategies that might help patients to manage this chronic, disabling, and often painful condition more successfully. Of course, these forms of treatment and management offer much less scope than drugs for commercial exploitation so are too often ignored.

How many other fields of therapeutic research would, if evaluated in this way, reveal similar mismatches between the questions about treatment effects that matter to patients and clinicians, and those that researchers are addressing? Other examples[85, 86, 87] lead us to suspect that mismatch is the rule rather than the exception. Minor changes in drug formulation rarely lead to the drugs having substantially new, more useful effects, yet these types of studies dominate research into treatments for arthritis and for other disorders. What a waste of resources!

Clearly this situation is unsatisfactory, so how has it come about? One reason is that what gets studied by researchers is distorted by external factors.[88] The pharmaceutical industry, for example, does research for its primary need – to fulfil its overriding responsibility to shareholders, not to patients and clinicians. Businesses are driven by large markets – such as women wondering whether to use hormone replacement therapy, or people who are depressed, anxious, unhappy, or in pain. Yet only rarely in recent decades has this commercially targeted approach led to important new treatments, even for 'mass market' disorders. Rather, within groups of drugs, industry has produced many very similar compounds – so-called 'me-too' drugs. This is reminiscent of the days when the only bread available in supermarkets was endless variations on the white sliced loaf. Hardly surprising, then, that the pharmaceutical industry spends more on marketing than on research.

But how does industry persuade prescribers to use these new products rather than existing, less expensive alternatives? A common strategy is to commission numerous small research projects showing that the new drugs are better than giving nothing at all, while not doing any research to find out whether the new drugs are better than the existing ones. Regrettably, industry has little difficulty in finding doctors who are willing to enrol their patients in this fruitless enterprise. And the same doctors often end up

'In British Columbia most (80%) of the increase in drug expenditure between 1996 and 2003 was explained by the use of new, patented drug products that did not offer substantial improvements on less expensive alternatives available before 1990. The rising cost of using these me-too drugs at prices far exceeding those of time tested competitors deserves careful scrutiny. Approaches to drug pricing such as those used in New Zealand may enable savings that could be diverted towards other healthcare needs. For example, $350m (26% of total expenditure on prescription drugs) would have been saved in British Columbia if half of the me-too drugs consumed in 2003 were priced to compete with older alternatives. This saving could pay the fees of more than a thousand new doctors.

Given that the list of top 20 drugs in global sales includes newly patented versions of drugs in long established categories . . . me-too drugs probably dominate spending trends in most developed countries.'

Morgan SG, Bassett KL, Wright JM, *et al.* 'Breakthrough' drugs and growth in expenditure on prescription drugs in Canada. *British Medical Journal* 2005;331:815-6.

promoting the products studied in this way.[89] Drug licensing authorities often make the problem worse by insisting that new drugs should be compared with placebos, rather than with existing effective treatments.

Commentaries in prestigious medical journals such as *The Lancet*[90] have drawn attention to the perverse incentives now driving some of those involved in clinical research, and the increasingly dubious relationships between universities and industry. One editorialist in the *New England Journal of Medicine*[91] asked bluntly 'Is academic medicine for sale?'

However, commercial priorities are not the only perverse influences on patterns of biomedical research that disregard the interests of patients. Many people within universities and research funding organisations believe that improvements in health are most likely to stem from attempts to unravel basic mechanisms of disease. So, they do research in laboratories and with animals. Although such basic research is unquestionably needed, there is precious little evidence to support this bias towards it.[92, 93] Yet the consequence has been a massive outpouring of laboratory research that has not been properly evaluated to see how relevant it is to patients.

One reason for this distortion is the hype surrounding the hoped-for clinical advances that basic research might offer. Fifty years after the structure of DNA was discovered, for example, the cacophony of claims about the ensuing potential benefits for healthcare is almost deafening.

Writing a light-hearted article for a Christmas edition of the *British Medical Journal*, two researchers created a spoof company called HARLOT plc to provide a series of services for trial sponsors. For example:

'We can guarantee positive results for the manufacturers of dodgy drugs and devices who are seeking to increase their market shares, for health professional guilds who want to increase the demand for their unnecessary diagnostic and therapeutic services, and for local and national health departments who are seeking to implement irrational and self serving health policies . . . for dodgy "me too" drugs . . . as long as your "me too" drug isn't a lot worse than a sip of triple distilled water, [our E-Zee-Me-Too Protocol team] can guarantee you a positive trial.'

To their astonishment, the authors received some apparently serious inquiries about the amazing HARLOT plc portfolio.

Sackett DL, Oxman AD. HARLOT plc: an amalgamation of the world's two oldest professions.
British Medical Journal 2003;327:1442-5.

Yet, as one geneticist has observed, 'for twenty years geneticists have issued a stream of promises about what they will achieve. Few have been fulfilled, and some never will be.'[94] There is no way of bypassing responsibly the need for well-designed research in patients to test the therapeutic theories derived from basic research. And, all too often, such theories are never followed through to see if they do have any relevance for patients. More than a decade after researchers identified the genetic defect leading to cystic fibrosis, people with the condition are still asking when they will see dividends to their health resulting from the discovery (see Chapter 2).

BETTER RESEARCH

Even when research may seem relevant to patients, researchers often appear to overlook patients' concerns when they design their studies. In a telling illustration, lung cancer doctors were asked to put themselves in the position of patients and to consider whether they would consent to participate in each of six lung cancer trials for which they might, as patients, be eligible. Between 36 and 89 per cent of them said that they would not participate – presumably because the doctors did not think the questions being addressed in the research were important enough.[95]

Similarly, in clinical trials in psoriasis – a chronic and disabling skin condition that affects about two out of every 100 people in the UK – patients' interests have been poorly represented. The Psoriasis Association found that researchers persisted in using a largely discredited scoring system in many studies to assess the effects of various treatments. Among its deficiencies, the scoring system concentrates on measures such as total area of skin affected and thickness of the lesions, whereas patients, not surprisingly, are more troubled by lesions on the face, palms and soles, and genitals.[96]

So, has anything improved in the decade since the *British Medical Journal* editorial drew attention to the scandal of poor medical research? Happily yes. Stimulated by surveys revealing the poor quality of many reports of clinical trials, reporting standards have been developed and applied (see Chapter 3). Such standards make clear, for example, exactly how many patients have been asked to participate in a study, how many declined the invitation, and the results according to the various treatment groups selected at the outset. But there is still a long way to go to improve: (a) the choice of questions being addressed in research; (b) the way that these questions are formulated to ensure that the outcomes of treatments chosen for assessment are those that patients regard as important; and (c) the information made available to patients.

Belatedly, some researchers have begun to realise the importance of working with patients, carers, and the public to find out about their experiences of illness and healthcare. Social scientists are increasingly integral members of research teams testing treatments. As a result, formal methods of exploring these aspects of illness have been developed and new ways of integrating this evidence with traditional approaches are being introduced. When patients are invited to join clinical trials where the questions have been planned in partnership with researchers, they will

---

PSORIASIS PATIENTS POORLY SERVED BY RESEARCH

'Few trials involved comparison of different options or looked at long-term management. The duration of studies is unconvincingly brief in the context of a disease of potentially near life-long chronicity. We seem to know reliably only that our treatments are better than nothing at all. Tellingly, researchers have completely ignored patient experience, views, preferences, or satisfactions.'

Jobling R. Therapeutic research into psoriasis: patients' perspectives, priorities and interests. In: Rawlins M, Littlejohns P, eds. *Delivering quality in the NHS 2005*. Abingdon: Radcliffe Publishing Ltd, pp53-56.

be more likely to identify with the need to reduce uncertainty.[97, 98, 99, 100, 101, 102] To explore the feasibility and acceptability of a proposed trial, preliminary studies with groups of patients can be useful. Such studies may highlight shortcomings in the design plans; or help to define outcomes that are more relevant; or even suggest that the concept is a nonstarter. This can save a lot of time, money, and frustration. Preparatory work done for a clinical trial in men with localised prostate cancer (see Chapter 7) provided some interesting lessons. The preliminary studies revealed how the research design could be improved by careful consideration of the terms used by clinicians to describe the trial's purpose and the treatment options. When cancer has not spread beyond the prostate gland itself, the uncertainty is whether it is preferable simply to monitor patients regularly or to advise surgery or radiotherapy. Studies have shown that many older men who have died of heart disease, stroke, or other causes have – incidentally – localised prostate cancer that had never affected their health. Yet the preparatory work for the trial revealed that clinicians clearly had difficulty in discussing the uncertainty about the value of treating this symptomless condition. Similarly, they were hesitant to describe the treatment options equally.

The clinicians also unknowingly used words that patients misinterpreted. For example, when describing the monitoring arm of the trial they often used the phrase 'watchful waiting'. Patients tended to interpret this as 'no treatment' – as if doctors would 'watch while I die'. Consequently the researchers replaced this by the term 'active monitoring', with a detailed description of what this would entail in terms of regular surveillance. Additionally, fearing that this arm of the trial might prove unpopular, clinicians often left talking about it until last. Moreover, they unwittingly created unease by the phrase they used to suggest there was a good chance of surviving beyond 10 years. What they said was: 'the majority of men with prostate cancer will be alive 10 years later'. This was interpreted, more negatively, as 'some men will be dead in 10 years' rather than 'most men with prostate cancer live long lives even with the disease'.

Thus, in the trial, sensitive exploration of patients' views in preliminary studies, rather than the imposition of trialists' design ideas, led to an acceptable and feasible way to compare the treatment options. An acceptable study seems likely to recruit in a shorter time, thereby identifying the good and bad effects of treatments more quickly for patients and those treating them.

RESEARCH FOR THE RIGHT REASONS

With the lion's share of biomedical research funding invested in laboratory and animal studies, there is now a funding crisis in research studies that are likely to yield evidence more immediately relevant to patients.[103, 104] Consequently, the pharmaceutical industry's financial clout calls too many of the shots when it comes to deciding which questions about the effects of treatments will be studied. Academics, and the institutions they work in, too often take part in trials addressing questions of interest to industry's agenda because industry can pay them thousands of pounds for each patient recruited. Sometimes these 'bounty payments' are used to bolster the institutions' funds; but not infrequently individual doctors benefit from them financially.

Some of the other reward systems within universities also lead to research being done for the wrong reasons. As a former editor of the *New England Journal of Medicine* noted: 'large-scale multi-institutional clinical trials provide less opportunity for authorship than individual or small-group research'.[105] Authorship of research reports is highly prized within universities as a condition of personal academic advancement and a measure of institutional success and continued funding. As a result, researchers and the institutions in which they work regard multicentre, collaborative research projects – which are often published in the name of a group – as a threat to individual recognition and kudos. So, studies continue to be done by individual researchers and small teams and are often not big enough to yield reliable results that are important to patients.

And within the UK, the university funding allocation system from government actually encourages this tendency, thus reinforcing a system that serves academic interests rather than those of patients. One senior neurologist who has done more than most to help stroke patients ruefully pointed out: 'the real credit for thinking up, designing and then running RCTs [randomised controlled trials] is often lost in collaborative group authorship, necessary as this is to acknowledge the contribution of the many people involved. A senior university official once castigated me for not being cited enough; but as a competitive basic scientist-businessman he had no idea of my part in a trial, lost as I was in the (group) authorship'.[106]

This distorted research agenda raises worrying questions, not only about the research that does get done and reported, but also about the research that does not get done at all. The 'opportunity cost' of these tendencies is substantial – many questions about the effects of treatments intended to improve health are not being addressed because they do not interest either the commercial sector or universities.

For example, there was controversy for nearly a century about how to control convulsions (fits) in women experiencing eclampsia – a life-threatening complication of pregnancy (see Chapter 5) which is associated with the deaths of an estimated 50,000 women every year. There is no commercial interest in this question for two reasons: (a) most of the women who die from the condition live in developing countries, and (b) one of the treatments – magnesium sulphate, long used in Epsom salts – offers no scope for commercial profits. There was little academic interest in the controversy because it can only be addressed satisfactorily in a large, international collaborative study – and that meant that the identity of individual researchers and institutions would not be prominent in the shared credit appropriate for the work.

A study comparing different drugs for controlling eclamptic convulsions was eventually publicly funded in the 1990s by the UK Overseas Development Administration and the World Health Organisation. It showed that the cheapest drug was substantially more effective than more expensive alternatives.[107] The study report contains a telling comment: 'From magnesium sulphate first being suggested for women with eclampsia (in 1906) to the introduction of diazepam (in 1968), a possible 33 million women would have had an eclamptic convulsion and 3 million of them may have died. Up to 1987, when phenytoin was introduced, a further 9 million women possibly had a convulsion and one million died.' Clearly the price of distorted research priorities can be very high indeed.

MAGNESIUM FOR PREVENTING AND TREATING ECLAMPSIA

'Seven years ago, a study dubbed by one commentator as the most important obstetric randomised trial of the 20th century showed that, of three common approaches to controlling eclamptic convulsions, magnesium sulphate was the most effective. The Collaborative Eclampsia Trial was a landmark in several respects: the participation of 1,687 women and their carers in 27 hospitals in nine developing countries achieved more than all the small-scale poorly controlled investigations over the previous 50 years, mainly in the countries in which only 1% of the world's cases of eclampsia occur. The report of the trial had a dramatic effect on practice in the UK, one of the countries in which magnesium sulphate had not been widely used by obstetricians. The trial is a good example of how collaborations between the developing and developed worlds can lead to improved clinical practice.'

Sheth S, Chalmers I. Magnesium for preventing and treating eclampsia: time for international action. *Lancet* 2002;359:1872-3.

Sometimes systematic reviews of existing research help to expose ignorance about the effects of widely used treatments which are of little commercial or academic interest. One such review explored whether steroids given to people with brain injury as a result of physical trauma increased or decreased their chances of survival. The completed review showed that it was unclear one way or the other.[108] Failure to resolve this uncertainty during the decades that the treatment had been used in hundreds of thousands of people had substantial human costs. When the necessary international collaborative study of steroids was eventually done, it revealed that the treatment had probably been killing thousands of patients with brain injury.[109] Yet this study faced some opposition from industry and some university researchers. Why? They were engaged in commercial trials assessing the effects of expensive new drugs – so-called neuroprotective agents – on outcome measures of questionable importance to patients, and they did not wish to face competition for participants.

This example illustrates the crucial importance of addressing questions which are of no interest to industry or universities: failure to do so can result in patients being harmed. There is currently inadequate funding in the UK for clinical trials done independently of industry. This has been recognised by the House of Commons Select Committee on Health,[110] and it has been reflected in the creation of the UK Clinical Research Collaboration (www.ukcrc.org), and new strategies within the Medical Research Council,[111] the NHS Research and Development Programme,[112] and some medical research charities. It remains to be seen how well these new arrangements address patients' and clinicians' unanswered questions about the effects of treatment.

Another reason for tackling these unanswered questions is to help ensure that the precious resources available for healthcare are not being wasted. For example, human albumin solution given as an intravenous drip was introduced during the 1940s to resuscitate burned and other critically ill patients. Theory suggested that albumin should reduce their chances of dying. Amazingly, this theory was not subjected to fair tests until the 1990s. At that point, a systematic review of the relevant controlled trials could find no evidence that human albumin solution reduced the risk of death. What the review showed, in fact, was that if albumin had any effect on death risk it was to increase it.[113]

The findings in this review prompted doctors in Australia and New Zealand to get together to do the first sufficiently large fair comparison of human albumin solution with saline (salt water), an alternative resuscitation fluid.[114] This study – which should have been done half a century earlier – could find no evidence that albumin was better than salt water. Since albumin is about 20 times more expensive than saline, billions of pounds' worth of healthcare resources worldwide will have been wasted over the past 50 years or so.

7

IMPROVING TESTS OF TREATMENTS IS EVERYBODY'S BUSINESS

In the preceding chapters we have shown how much time, money, and effort can be wasted in doing bad or unnecessary research into the effects of treatments – research that does not, and never will, answer questions that matter to patients. We have also outlined some of the problems that can prevent steady progress in grappling with the inevitable uncertainties that beset research into treatments.

In Chapter 1 we described how some new treatments have had harmful effects that were unexpected whereas the hoped-for effects of others have failed to materialise, and in Chapter 2 we highlighted the fact that many commonly used treatments and screening tests have not been

---

LIFTING THE FOG OF UNCERTAINTY

'Only when the public finally grasps how little reliable knowledge exists will it have the motivation to become actively involved in prioritising the research agenda. Ultimately improvement in clinical care and patients' outcomes will come from conducting the right kind of research, research that is of importance in the real world, as advocated in the recently established James Lind Alliance. Acknowledging uncertainties and informing patients about them is a key strategy for improving healthcare and lifting the fog from the practice of medicine.'

Djulbegovic B. Lifting the fog of uncertainty from the practice of medicine.
British Medical Journal 2004;329:1419-20.

'Who has the power to see that research questions actually address the greatest needs of patients in all their misery and diversity? Why aren't the most relevant questions being asked? Who is currently setting the questions? Who should be? Who shall direct this prioritisation? Patients are best able to identify the health topics most relevant to them and to inform their comfort, care, and quality of life, as well as its quantity. The patients are the David, who must load their slings against the Goliaths of the pharmaceutical companies who need evidence to market goods and make profits, and trialists who are driven by curiosity, the need to secure research money, professional acclaim, and career development. Profit, scientific inquiry, grant money, and research papers are acceptable only if the central motivation is the good of patients. Independent patients and organisations that advocate good quality research should ready their sling, carefully choose their stone, take aim, and conquer.'

Refractor. Patients' choice: David and Goliath. *Lancet* 2001;358:768.

adequately evaluated. In Chapter 3 we outlined the basis for fair testing of treatments, emphasising the importance of paying attention to reducing potential biases and taking account of the play of chance. In Chapter 4 we described some of the numerous uncertainties that pervade almost every aspect of healthcare, and in Chapter 5 we contrasted the key differences between good, bad, and unnecessary research into the effects of treatments. In Chapter 6 we pointed out how much of the research that is done is distorted by commercial and academic priorities and fails to address issues that are likely to make a real difference to the well-being of patients. We hope we have convinced you that better testing of treatments in the future should come from productive partnerships between researchers and patients.

So, how could patients improve research – both what is researched, and how studies are undertaken? In Chapter 6 we described how investigators in Bristol, working with focus groups of patients, rheumatologists, physiotherapists, and general practitioners, identified the discrepancies between the research that was being done into osteoarthritis of the knee and what was needed by those with the disease and the people treating them. Clinicians and patients were plainly tired of research on drugs. Instead, they wanted evaluation of other interventions: physiotherapy and surgery; educational and coping strategies.[115] The Bristol research also showed how facilitated discussion among groups of patients and health professionals could reveal what their priorities were, and which uncertainties about the effects of treatments mattered most to them and should be addressed.

But do the voices of patients and the public really count in the conduct of healthcare research? Happily, the formerly closed world of medicine is opening its doors to admit fresh ideas and former 'outsiders'. Paternalism is steadily diminishing. There is increasing support for involving patients as partners in the research process. And there is accumulating evidence from questionnaire surveys;[116] systematic reviews of research reports;[117] and reports of individual trials[118] that involvement of patients and the public can contribute to improving tests of treatments. Patients have experience that can enhance deliberations and provide insights. Their first-hand knowledge can shed valuable light on the way in which people react to illness and how this affects choice of treatments.

Roles are evolving[119] to accommodate various ways of enabling patients and the public to work with health professionals to improve the testing of healthcare interventions. This is happening across the spectrum of research activities:

- formulation of questions to be addressed
- design of projects, including selection of outcomes
- project management
- development of patient information leaflets
- analysis and interpretation of results, and
- dissemination and implementation of findings.

How has this come about? In Chapter 2 we showed, for example, how the treatment excesses formerly imposed on women with breast cancer led to challenges and changes, both from a new breed of clinician researchers and then from patients. Doctors and patients collaborated to secure the research evidence that met both rigorous scientific standards and the needs of women. When women challenged the practice of radical mastectomy they signalled that they were concerned about more than eradication of cancer: they demanded a say in the tactics employed to deal with the disease.

Today, there are moves away from clinicians imposing treatments and research on patients. It is no longer acceptable to measure 'success' by patients' unquestioning compliance with the treatments prescribed. A better way to provide treatments that patients identify as important and relevant to their care is to encourage shared responsibility for making decisions, for taking medicines, and for testing health interventions of all kinds.

'In terms of involvement in decision making ('who chooses'), patients most prefer a consultation in which they contribute but do not have sole respons-ibility for the decision taken (shared model). Least preferred are consultations where the doctor alone makes the decisions (paternalistic).'

Thornton H, Edwards A, Elwyn G. Evolving the multiple roles of 'patients' in health-care research: reflections after involvement in a trial of shared decision-making. *Health Expectations* 2003;6:189-97.

PATIENTS NEED INFORMATION

Patients in partnerships in healthcare need access to good quality, under-standable information – whether in the one-to-one relationship of a consultation, or when considering whether they should join a trial, or as members of research teams. Without this, there is little prospect of meaningful dialogue and real patient involvement.

Patients regularly complain about lack of information. Although some prefer not to have detailed information about their illness and treatment options and to leave things entirely to their professional advisers, many are keen to learn more. They want to know and understand how the results of treatment tests have a bearing on them personally. For them, openness and transparency are essential. They need the assurance that everyone knows what tests of treatments are going on; that results are published, whether 'positive' or 'negative'; that systematic reviews of all the relevant evidence are undertaken and kept up to date; and that adverse effects are not covered up. Clearly, patients need to be sure that researchers know what has already been done before embarking on new research: as we have outlined in earlier chapters, patients have suffered when researchers have not bothered to find out what has gone before.

One early example of patient support for and involvement in proper evaluation relates to the introduction of chorionic villus sampling in the 1980s. Chorionic villus sampling is a way of diagnosing abnormalities in the fetus at an earlier stage of pregnancy than is possible with amniocent-esis. Despite the real possibility that the new technique would be more likely than amniocentesis to provoke miscarriage, it had been taken up by women at very high risk (1 in 4) of carrying a fetus with a severe inherited blood disorder. For these women and their families, the wish to avoid bringing into the world a child who would suffer pain and an early death outweighed the potential risk that the new technique might provoke the miscarriage of a normal fetus.

A medical researcher who underwent a few blood tests after an episode of back pain was told he had some results that were not clear cut but were somewhat worrying. Over the next few years the diagnosis of a type of blood cancer (myeloma) became clear. He reflected on what had happened, including the unavailability of evidence:

'What are the lessons? Firstly, that as a patient I felt even more strongly about what I've been fighting for throughout my career. Research results should be easily accessible to people who need to make decisions about their own health. The delay in the analysis of the four randomised controlled trials struck me as a case in point. Why was I forced to make my decision knowing that information was somewhere but not available? Was the delay because the results were less exciting than expected? Or because in the evolving field of myeloma research there are now new exciting theories (or drugs) to look at? How far can we tolerate the butterfly behaviour of researchers, moving on to the next flower well before the previous one has been fully exploited? Unfortunately this is possible in a world where clinical research has become dominated by commercial interests. When you are a patient you wonder how (we) researchers can keep forgetting the principle that the priority should be collaboration for better hypotheses, not competition.'

Liberati A. An unfinished trip through uncertainties.
British Medical Journal 2004;328:531.

However, the balance was very different for other women who were much less likely – between 1 in 50 and 1 in 200, for example – to have an affected fetus. For them it was important to know whether the more invasive test – chorionic villus sampling – was indeed more likely than amniocentesis to provoke a miscarriage or some other problem. Consequently, the Medical Research Council backed an international collaboration to address these questions. This initiative was supported widely by the press. In the UK, for example, most journalists applauded the planned research and emphasised the importance of careful evaluation before deciding whether new medical techniques should be adopted more widely.

An example of irresponsible advice offered by a clinician in a letter to The Guardian newspaper was that women should demand the new, inadequately tested procedure straight away. This provoked a stern response from the co-ordinator of the Maternity Alliance, an umbrella organisation of pressure groups. She strongly defended the need for the study.

In what was probably an unprecedented move to promote a randomised trial at the time, a lay pressure group, the Association for Improvements in the Maternity Services, convened a meeting of interested voluntary organisations and patient groups to encourage them to give public support to the Medical Research Council's proposals. Representatives of these groups helped to draft the information leaflet for potential participants in the trial, and the leaflet made clear that seven lay organisations had formally and publicly endorsed the study. Significantly, these lay groups also agreed that the trial organisers should try to ensure that no woman would be offered the new technique outside the study unless she had previously conceived a genetically damaged child.[120]

Early activists in the breast cancer field also realised that they should speak up and challenge the status quo – and that to do so they needed accurate information. First they set about educating themselves so that they could become effective. Then they set about educating others. For example, Rose Kushner, an American breast cancer patient and freelance writer, challenged the traditional authoritarian physician/patient relationship and the need for radical surgery in the early 1970s.[121] She wrote a book based on her thorough review of evidence of the effects of radical mastectomy. By the end of the decade, her influence and acceptability were such that she worked with the US National Cancer Institute reviewing proposals for new research.[122]

In the UK, Betty Westgate's unhappy experience when she was diagnosed with breast cancer led her to set up the Mastectomy Association in the 1970s. This was the forerunner of Breast Cancer Care, which is now a flourishing organisation with branches in England, Scotland and Wales.[123, 124] Breast Cancer Care helps thousands of women seeking information and support. Another cancer patient, Vicky Clement-Jones, set up CancerBACUP as a national charity, to provide not only practical advice and emotional support to patients, but good quality information on treatment and research. Today, CancerBACUP and their cancer specialist nurses provide this service for nearly 50,000 people each year.

People with HIV/AIDS in the USA in the late 1980s were another exceptionally well-informed and well-organised group. They were politically geared to defend their interests against the establishment, paving the way for patients to participate in the design of trials. This involvement ultimately led to a choice of treatment options offered to patients in the trials and flexible designs to encourage participation. This example was

---

HELPING TO INFLUENCE FUTURE RESEARCH

'It is essential that cancer research takes into account the needs and interests of the people it is trying to help. Cancer specialists are usually aware of the gaps in their understanding of the diagnosis and treatment of cancer, but patients, their families and friends may see other aspects of their care that need further research.'

CancerBACUP. Understanding cancer research trials (clinical trials).
London: CancerBACUP, 2003.

followed in the early 1990s in the UK when an AIDS patient group was involved in studies at the Chelsea and Westminster Hospital, London: the patients helped to design study protocols.[125]

These AIDS activists made trialists sit up: what some researchers had viewed as havoc caused by organised patient groups was in fact a legitimate challenge to the trialists' interpretation of uncertainty. Until then, the researchers' approach had overlooked the patients' preferred outcomes. On the other hand, patients came to appreciate the dangers of making hasty judgements about the effects of new drugs and of demanding release of a 'promising' new AIDS drug before it had been evaluated rigorously. The researchers may have remonstrated that 'compassionate release' of new drugs in this way had merely prolonged the agony of uncertainty for current and future patients. However, the patients countered that it ultimately hastened the understanding of both patients and researchers about the need for unhurried, controlled evaluations of treatments within trials, designed jointly, and taking account of the needs of both parties.[126]

In the 1990s, one AIDS trial in particular provided a very special illustration of the importance of patient involvement. This was at a time when the drug zidovudine had recently been introduced for the treatment of AIDS. In patients with advanced disease there was good evidence of a beneficial effect. The obvious next question was whether use of zidovudine earlier in the course of infection might delay disease progression and further improve survival. So, trials were begun in both the USA and

Europe to test this possibility. The US trial was stopped early when a possible but still uncertain beneficial effect was found. With active participation and agreement of patient representatives, and despite the US results, the European trial continued to a clear endpoint. The result was very different: zidovudine used early in the course of infection did not appear to confer any benefit. The only clear effects of the drug in these circumstances were its unwanted side-effects.[127]

Regrettably, the lessons from the HIV/AIDS experience have not been learned in some other fields that present similar dilemmas. The rare diseases caused by prions – such as human versions of 'mad cow disease' – tend to strike down young people, and they are often rapidly fatal. Yet desperate attempts by relatives to access drugs that may help patients with these horrible conditions may actually delay the identification of treatments that do more good than harm. The father of one young man with prion disease learned through the internet that a drug which had never before been used in human beings to treat these conditions had shown some evidence of benefit in rodent experiments in Japan. As the drug was not licensed for use in human prion disease (it has to be given directly into the brain and can cause bleeding there), the desperate father went to the High Court to ask that it be made available for his son. The judge concluded that although use of the treatment 'cannot be regarded as a research project, there would be an opportunity to learn, for the first time, the possible effects of PPS (pentosan polysulphate) [the unlicensed drug] on patients with vCJD [variant Creutzfeldt Jakob disease, one of the prion diseases]'. The judge's words reveal a worrying lack of understanding; she did not seem to realise that poorly controlled experimentation was likely to delay the discovery of treatments that can be helpful in prion disease.[128] She could have made her judgement conditional on a requirement that careful records would be made of treatment and progress of this patient, and the other patients who subsequently went to the High Court seeking a similar ruling. Had she done so, we would not remain as ignorant as we now are about the possible effects of this unevaluated treatment.

Even more recently, a patient with early breast cancer challenged the decision of the NHS not to give her the new drug Herceptin (trastuzumab). The Secretary of State for Health intervened and the NHS caved in. Herceptin appears to benefit some patients with advanced disease, but also seems to cause heart failure. It has not been sufficiently tested in early stages of the disease, and might ultimately prove to do more harm than good. It is too early to say.[129]

JEOPARDISING FAIR TESTS OF TREATMENTS

Involving patients in research is clearly not a panacea. For example, although a survey of researchers revealed some very positive experiences resulting from involving patients in clinical trials, it also laid bare some very real problems.[130] Many of these seemed to arise from patients' understandable lack of knowledge about how research is done and funded.

One of our aims in writing this book is to increase general knowledge about the principles of testing treatments and how reliable evidence of treatment effects is obtained. In this way, we hope we can assist patients who would like to help improve the quality of such evidence to do so more effectively. As we emphasised in Chapter 3, it is fundamentally important to equip patients with an awareness of how biases and the play of chance can mislead.

Patients may sometimes actually jeopardise fair tests of treatments if they do not understand the general principles of carrying out research and take these issues into account. Like the father of the young man with vCJD, desperate circumstances sometimes provoke desperate efforts to access treatments that have not been adequately evaluated and may do more harm than good, even to patients who are dying. We have already referred to the way that lobbying by patients and their advocates for 'compassionate' release of 'promising' new drug treatments for AIDS had its downside: it delayed the identification of treatments directed at outcomes that mattered to patients.

This is not the only such example. In the mid-1990s, interferons were introduced to treat patients with the relapsing-remitting form of multiple sclerosis on the basis of very scant evidence of benefit. In 2001 independent researchers carried out a systematic review of the evidence from controlled trials of these drugs,[131] every one of which had been organised and analysed by the manufacturers. The results of this review suggested that, although interferons reduced the frequency of relapses a little, there was no evidence that they affected the sustained progression of disability such as the need for walking aids or a wheelchair.

Because the annual cost of treating each patient with an interferon was over £10,000, the National Institute for Health and Clinical Excellence (NICE) – the organisation that assesses the cost-effectiveness of treatments for the National Health Service – concluded that using these drugs, and another one called glatiramer, would not be a responsible use of limited resources. Many patients with this debilitating disease, and especially the organisations lobbying on their behalf, were outraged. They were angry that the National Health Service could deny patients drugs that appeared to hold out some hope. Yet did they fully realise the extent to which the available evidence was far from convincing? It was based on partial release of the relevant research results, outcome measures of dubious relevance, and follow-up over only two or three years in a disease that usually lasts at least two decades.

The government caved in under the pressure. The Department of Health and the manufacturers developed a 10-year strategy to provide the drugs. But this effectively ended the possibility of learning whether they are helpful to patients. Worse still, because interferons had now become the accepted standard treatment for the disease, independent studies of alternative ways of helping patients had suddenly become prohibitively expensive. Why? Because clinicians and patients claimed that it had become unethical to compare any new treatment against placebos: new treatments had to be compared with the costly interferons.

ASSESSING DRUGS FOR MULTIPLE SCLEROSIS

1. NICE has announced that neither interferon beta nor glatiramer can be recommended for multiple sclerosis in the NHS.

2. The Department of Health plans to make these drugs available through a risk sharing scheme that is scientifically unsound and impractical.

3. Randomised trials suggest that azathioprine (which is 20 times cheaper) may be just as effective.

4. The long term effectiveness of these drugs is unknown.

5. Government money would be better spent on a long term randomised trial comparing interferon beta or glatiramer with azathioprine and no treatment.

Sudlow CLM, Counsell CE. Problems with UK government's risk sharing scheme for assessing drugs for multiple sclerosis. *British Medical Journal* 2003;326:388-92.

In multiple sclerosis, where industry-funded trials have all but elim-
inated independent academic initiatives, progress in treating the disease
may actually have been impeded – an unsatisfactory outcome by any
measure.

There is another important aspect of this sorry tale – how substantial
financial vested interests have prevented the proper testing of interferons
for multiple sclerosis. Drug companies sell interferons and some neurologists and other clinicians are paid by the drug companies to promote them.
Then there are the neurologists who use expensive brain scans to examine
patients on the unproven assumption that what they see in these images is
a valid way of monitoring the progress of the disease in terms relevant to
patients. This approach has been heavily promoted by industry. In spite of
the lack of evidence that these scans are useful in monitoring the progression of multiple sclerosis, many neurologists maintain that they must
be used in all clinical trials of treatments for the disease. Whereas industry
can meet and pass on to its customers the substantial costs (as much as
£2,000 per scan) of these unvalidated investigations, these costs are a
further obstacle facing those who wish to see studies done independently
of industry.

Another less well known conflict of interest exists in the relationship
between the patients' organisations and the pharmaceutical industry. Most
patients' organisations are poor, volunteer-based, and have little independent funding. Grants from and joint projects with pharmaceutical
companies can help them grow and be more influential, but can also
distort and misrepresent patients' agendas, including their research agendas. In some cases patient organisations have been set up by drug companies to lobby on behalf of their products. For instance, one of the
companies that makes interferon, which was subsequently taken to task
by the Medicines Control Agency, formed a new patient group 'Action for
Access' in an attempt to get the NHS to provide interferons for multiple
sclerosis.[132, 133] The message heard by patient groups from all of this
publicity was that interferons were effective but too expensive, when the
real issue was whether the drugs had any useful effects – and in a disease
characterised by false dawns for a century. Even now, some 16 years after
the first interferon trial began, there are still no meaningful long-term
data.

Not only is there serious doubt about whether new drugs for multiple
sclerosis have any effects of real importance to patients, some appear to
have very serious side-effects. In the USA, the Food and Drug Administration approved the biological drug Tysabri (natalizumab) on the basis of
only 12 months' data. The impact of this extraordinary decision was short-
lived: the company withdrew their product when two cases of a very rare

'The pharmaceutical industry does not donate money to charities for altruistic reasons. It is not allowed [in Europe] to advertise prescription drugs to patients [directly], but it knows that patient groups are often a strong lobby and have power to influence government and the NHS.

'Patients trust medical charities and expect their information to be unbiased and uninfluenced by the charity's funding sources. Charities accepting industry funding should declare it as a conflict of interest to enable patients to question their independence and that of the information they provide and seek further information from more independent sources.

'Arthritis Care launched a campaign for the wider prescribing of a new COX-2 inhibitor based on misleading positive results six months into a 12 month study. It did not declare that their campaign was funded by the drug manufacturers Pharmacia and Pfizer.

'The Impotence Association campaigns for wider prescription of Viagra and receives funding from Pfizer, whose logo appears on the association's website. Diabetes UK received around £1m from 11 pharmaceutical companies manufacturing diabetes drugs but this is not mentioned in the annual report.

'The lack of acknowledgement of sums of this magnitude leads people to be suspicious. Why not simply declare the true figures to the public? What is there to hide?'

Hirst J, Charities and patient groups should declare interests.
British Medical Journal 2003;326:1211.

fatal brain disease were reported among the small numbers of patients participating in a trial of the drug. Although this catastrophe was almost certainly caused by the new drug, and might have been even worse with longer exposure to it, patients and clinicians continued to clamour for it.

STEPS TO BETTER TESTING

In the previous section we drew attention to problems that can result from patients becoming involved in testing treatments, and ways in which they may unintentionally jeopardise fair tests. As with most things, good intentions do not guarantee that more good than harm will be done. Nevertheless, there are clear examples of the benefits of researchers and patients working together to improve the relevance and design of research. As a result, many researchers actively seek patients with whom they can collaborate.

An appropriate area for joint working is research designed to find out how to improve shared decision-making and risk-communication in general practice. For one of the trials with this aim, researchers worked with patients to develop the plans. First, they reviewed published reports to establish what aspects health professionals thought were important to patients during consultation with their doctors. Then they investigated patients' views directly by organising a series of focus groups involving both patients and citizens. They explored decision-making approaches, availability of information, and patients' perceptions of being involved in the decision. Rigorous research methods were used to establish what common ground there was between the published reports of professionals' and patients' priorities.

Patients who participated in the focus groups confirmed the importance to them of many of the outcomes that researchers had previously identified and used in publications – for example, perceived involvement in decisions and professional-patient agreement. However, the participants also identified a broader range of outcomes as being important: these included feeling respected as a 'player' who had made meaningful contributions when decisions were taken. They identified the need for accessible extra sources of information to help them assess the information given. Participants wanted the opportunity to involve others, such as family members, other professionals in the team, allied health professionals (nurses, counsellors), and voluntary or self-help support groups. They

---

COLLABORATION BETWEEN RESEARCHERS AND PATIENTS FOR MUTUAL BENEFIT

The publicly funded PRISM trial is a UK multicentre, randomised controlled trial comparing treatment strategies for Paget's disease of the bone. The National Association for the Relief of Paget's Disease (NARPD) is the only UK support group for sufferers of Paget's disease and has worked closely with the PRISM team from the outset. NARPD involvement is integral to the conduct of the trial and specific roles have included: peer-review; trial steering committee membership; provision of advice to participants, and promotion of the trial among Paget's disease patients.

Adapted from Langston A, McCallum M, Campbell M, Robertson C, Ralston S.
An integrated approach to consumer representation and involvement in a
multicentre randomized controlled trial. *Clinical Trials* 2005;2:80-7.

expressed strong preferences for continuity of care, including definite management plans and clear arrangements for review of treatment decisions, backed up by summary material or audio-taped information.[134]

In an example of the value of collaborative preparatory work, researchers explored with patients and potential patients some of the difficult issues involved in testing treatments given in an emergency. If therapies for acute stroke are to succeed, they need to be started as soon as possible after the stroke occurs. Because they were unsure of the best way to proceed, the researchers asked patients and carers to help them. They convened an exploratory meeting with a group of patients and health professionals, and conducted focus groups involving older people. As a result, plans for the trial were clarified and patients helped the researchers to draft and revise trial information leaflets.

This thorough preliminary research led to plans for a randomised controlled trial that were endorsed promptly by the research ethics committee. The focus group participants had recognised the ethical dilemmas of trying to obtain informed consent from someone with an acute illness which may well have left them confused, if not unconscious. They were able to suggest solutions that led to an acceptable trial design for all parties, and substantial improvements in the information leaflets.[135]

In Chapter 6, we described the importance of the preparatory work

---

THE IMPORTANCE OF PATIENT INVOLVEMENT IN PLANNING RESEARCH

Researchers got together groups of elderly people to think through the design of a new study into how to treat people suffering an acute stroke – at the point of actually having a stroke, patients, understandably, often cannot contribute their views. The researchers concluded that:

- Involvement of patients in the design of trials on stroke is valuable
- Comments from people who have not yet had a stroke, and from carers of those who have, can enable substantial improvements of trial information leaflets
- People support different consent approaches depending on the clinical state of the patient
- Patient involvement can be a very important part of the development of new randomised controlled trials

Adapted from Koops L, Lindley RI.
Thrombolysis for acute ischaemic stroke: consumer involvement in design of new
randomised controlled trial. *British Medical Journal* 2002;325:415-7.

with patients for a UK trial of treatments for localised prostate cancer. The researchers, for sound reasons, wanted to compare the effects of active monitoring with surgery or radiotherapy to reduce the uncertainty surrounding these therapies. Clearly these are widely dissimilar forms of treatment, so how would patients and their clinicians react to the proposed random allocation to one or other of these options? The researchers had no difficulty in identifying likely barriers that clinicians might face in trying to present the trial to patients. They could also imagine that patients would find it difficult to decide whether to enter the trial, especially because they would need to agree to be randomised to one of three such different treatments with different potential complications.

Against this background, the researchers developed a two-phase proposal: first a feasibility study and then use of the results to conduct the main trial. Findings from their first phase showed that the trial was feasible and that most men would agree to be recruited to a three-arm (active monitoring, surgery, or radiotherapy) study.[136]

HOW SHOULD PATIENTS AND THE PUBLIC BECOME INVOLVED?

There are numerous ways in which patients and the public can become involved in testing treatments. As we have already outlined, they may be the prime movers – the ones who identify the gaps in understanding and the need to find new ways of doing things. Their input may be facilitated by researchers; they may be involved in some stages of the work but not others; they may be involved from the moment of identification of a specific uncertainty that needs addressing through to dissemination and incorporation of the project's findings in an updated systematic review; and they may be involved in different ways within one project. Sometimes they initiate the work themselves. There is no hard and fast rule: the appropriateness of different strategies and approaches in a particular study will dictate those chosen. As the localised prostate cancer trial and the shared decision-making trial illustrated, methods are evolving all the time – even within the course of a project.

A systematic review of patient involvement in identifying and prioritising possible topics for research was published in 2004.[137] This report concluded that those in charge of research programmes now have adequate collective experience of involving patients to plan their research agendas by working directly or indirectly with the public. Research funding bodies often now ask research applicants to make clear how they plan to involve members of the public and patients in their proposals, and advise researchers where they can learn more about how to do this.

1. The roles of patients are agreed between the researchers and patients involved in the research.
2. Researchers budget appropriately for the costs of patient involvement in research.
3. Researchers respect the differing skills, knowledge and experience of patients.
4. Patients are offered training and personal support to enable them to be involved in research.
5. Researchers ensure that they have the necessary skills to involve patients in the research process.
6. Patients are involved in decisions about how participants in research are recruited and kept informed about the progress of the research.
7. Patient involvement is described in research reports.
8. Research findings are available to patients in formats and in language they can easily understand.

Adapted from Telford R, Boote JD, Cooper CL.
What does it mean to involve consumers successfully in NHS research?
A consensus study. *Health Expectations* 2004;7:209-20.

So, overall, involvement of patients and the public is coming of age. No longer are they to be ignored or merely included as a token gesture. As partners in research they can make for a better choice of research topics and for better conduct of the research itself. Although patients may sometimes inadvertently jeopardise fair testing of treatments, patients and researchers working together offer a powerful combination for reducing treatment uncertainties for the benefit of all.

KEY POINTS

- Patients and researchers working together offer a powerful combination for reducing treatment uncertainties for the benefit of all
- Patients can influence research on the effects of treatments
- Input from patients can lead to better research
- Patients sometimes inadvertently jeopardise fair testing of treatments
- To contribute effectively, patients need better general knowledge about research and readier access to information

8

BLUEPRINT FOR A REVOLUTION

We have no doubt about the contribution of medical research to better quality of life and longevity. Nevertheless, in this book we illustrate how the existing 'drivers' for research – commercial and academic – have not done enough to identify patients' priorities. Healthcare will always be full of uncertainties, of greater or lesser importance, and where better to address them than the NHS, in which all of us have a stake. So how do we bring about a revolution in which uncertainties in everyday healthcare are not dodged, but taken up as challenges; in which research to test treatments becomes a vital part of good healthcare?

Before outlining our blueprint for this revolution, let us give you a feeling for what we hope might happen in the routine setting of a general practice in future.

THE CASE OF MR JONES

Ifor Jones, a retired hill farmer in rural north Wales, has been much bothered by tiredness, and eventually decides to go and see his general practitioner. Ifor first checks when his daughter will be able to drive him the ten miles to the surgery, and then books an appointment to see the doctor. The doctor discusses Ifor's symptoms with him and examines him, and then takes some blood for tests and sends this to the local hospital for analysis. A few days later, the test results come back and they show that Ifor has a form of anaemia resulting from a lack of vitamin B12 (pernicious anaemia, see Chapter 4). The doctor telephones Ifor and asks him to come to see her again.

At the follow-up visit the doctor explains that the form of anaemia confirmed by the blood tests should respond very well to injections of vitamin B12, but she mentions that experts cannot agree whether injections are needed only every three months, or more frequently. Calling up the National Library for Health on her computer screen, the doctor shows Ifor a systematic review of controlled trials comparing different injection frequencies. This confirms that no one knows whether injections given more frequently than once every quarter might relieve tiredness more effectively.

The computer also draws their attention to some patient-friendly information about a controlled trial comparing different injection frequencies of vitamin B12 for pernicious anaemia. The study is being run by the NHS Research and Development Programme. It was started because several general practitioners and some patients had indicated through clinical question answering services that they wanted to know how frequently patients with pernicious anaemia should receive injections. Since organising repeat visits to the surgery for injections every month would be more inconvenient but might improve Ifor's symptoms more effectively, the doctor asks him whether he would consider participating in the trial.

When researchers and patients designed the trial to compare the effects of different treatment frequencies, the patients made sure that their most troublesome symptoms – for example, tiredness – would be assessed, alongside the standard blood tests for pernicious anaemia. Ifor and his doctor reckon that participating in the study will be very straightforward: no information will be required over and above that which the doctor would normally collect for monitoring the impact of the treatment. Furthermore, preliminary results of the study are expected within a year, which means that Ifor himself can be expected to benefit from the new evidence.

The doctor asks Ifor whether he would like to take the patient information leaflet home and think about whether to participate, but Ifor decides to sign up for the study there and then. The doctor enters Ifor's details in a password-protected, confidential section of the study website, and, within a few seconds, receives information from the study co-ordinating centre that Ifor has been randomly allocated to receive injections every three months.

Every quarter thereafter, the study co-ordinating centre sends text messages to the doctor's and Ifor's mobile phones, prompting them to answer some questions about Ifor's symptoms and signs, and to send further samples of blood to the laboratory. The laboratory then sends copies of the results to the study co-ordinating centre as well as to Ifor and his doctor.

A little over a year later, the doctor and Ifor receive initial results of the study. They take these into account in deciding whether they should continue with the three-monthly injection schedule, or opt for more frequent injections. Ifor and his doctor have thus contributed to reducing the uncertainty on a matter important to them both.

This illustration of a way to serve the interests of a patient who has vitamin B12-deficient anaemia, and those of a general practitioner uncertain about the relative merits of treatment options, highlights several points. Although effective treatments for this type of anaemia were identified nearly a century ago,[138] questions about how frequently to give vitamin B12 injections have gone unanswered because they were of scant interest to industry or academic researchers. Such questions will come to the fore only if recognised and addressed at the grass roots. In this particular example, little extra effort is needed beyond routine care to get the answer.

Our example refers to uncertainties about treatment effects on a chronic condition that can cause misery. However, the same basic approach should be followed to address uncertainties across the board – from life-threatening acute emergencies (such as acute stroke), to self-limiting but often annoying conditions like the common cold. What can we all do to ensure that the approach we have outlined becomes usual within the NHS?

OUR BLUEPRINT

Taken individually, none of the suggestions that follows is revolutionary, or even novel. Taken together and promoted jointly by patients and clinicians, our seven action points constitute a blueprint for a revolution in the use and testing of treatments.

1. Encourage honesty when there are uncertainties about the effects of treatments

Admitting uncertainty is often hard for health professionals, and it is sometimes not welcomed by patients. As a result, people are sometimes being given a false sense of security. If clinicians and patients are to work together successfully for more efficient assessment of treatment effects, both must be more ready to acknowledge that inadequately evaluated treatments can do substantial harm; they must become more familiar with the methods needed to obtain reliable evidence. We need to find out the best ways of making this happen.

2. Confront double standards on consent to treatment offered within and outside clinical trials

Clinicians who are prepared to admit uncertainties about the effects of treatments and address them in formal treatment comparisons are subject to more stringent rules for interacting with patients than are their colleagues. When there are uncertainties about treatment effects, participation in controlled trials or other methods of unbiased evaluation should be the norm. We should ensure that participation in research on treatment effects is not presented as a risky endeavour, implying that 'standard' practice is always effective and safe.

3. Increase knowledge about how to judge whether claims about treatment effects are trustworthy

A condition for change is greater public engagement with the ways in which bias and the play of chance can seriously distort evidence about the effects of treatments. One of the most important features of scientific investigation – recognising and minimising bias – can hardly be regarded as 'general knowledge'. We need more determined efforts to reduce these important gaps in understanding, and to make these concepts a routine part of education, from school age onwards.

4. Increase the capacity for preparing, maintaining, and disseminating systematic reviews of research evidence about the effects of treatments

Many of the answers to pressing questions about the effects of treatments can be readily addressed by systematically reviewing evidence that already exists, by keeping such reviews up to date, and by disseminating the results efficiently to professionals and patients. There is a long way to go before the messages from existing evidence are readily available in systematic reviews. We should urge the NHS to make this one of its prime goals, so that reliable information about the effects of treatments is synthesised and made readily accessible throughout the health service.

5. Tackle scientific misconduct and conflicts of interest within the clinical research community

Many people are astonished to find that researchers are not required to assess systematically what is known already when they seek funding and ethical approval for new research. The consequence is inevitable – poorly designed and frankly unnecessary research continues on a scale that is unacceptable on ethical as well as scientific grounds. We should press research funders and research ethics committees to ensure that researchers do not embark on new research of any kind without referring to systematic reviews of other relevant evidence. Furthermore, biased under-reporting of research is unethical. Researchers should be required to publish the results of all research to which patients have contributed, and to make clear what contribution the new evidence has made to the totality of relevant evidence.

6. Require industry to provide better, more complete, and more relevant evidence about the effects of treatment

In 2005, the House of Commons Health Committee published a hard-hitting report on the influence of the pharmaceutical industry.[139] Whenever the power and influence of the drug industry has been challenged in the past, the pharmaceutical giants have responded with near threats to withdraw their research and development activities from the UK and have issued dire warnings about the consequences for the UK economy. Successive governments have listened, capitulated, and done nothing to curb the industry's excesses. The Committee's recommendations should not be allowed to fall by the wayside. In particular, we should demand that all clinical trials are registered publicly at the outset, and that all the results are published in full on completion.

7. Identify and prioritise research addressing questions about the effects of treatments which are deemed important by patients and clinicians

The portfolios of research funders and academic institutions are dominated by basic research that is unlikely to benefit patients in the foreseeable future, and by research directed at maximising profits for industry. Applied research into questions that offer no potential to make money, yet matter to patients, has to fight for a toe-hold, even when it is publicly supported. We should see to it that the NHS does more to identify what questions patients and clinicians are asking about the effects of treatments, and that research funders take account of them in prioritising research to reduce these uncertainties.

IN CONCLUSION

A revolution in testing treatments is long overdue. If professionals and patients act together, the steps that we advocate are eminently practicable. You the readers should clamour for change – now.

Identify questions about the effects of treatments that are important to you.

Use the National Library for Health (www.library.nhs.uk) to see if there is reliable information from up-to-date systematic reviews.

If you can't find the information you need, ask NHS Direct to help you (www.nhsdirect.nhs.uk; Tel: 0845 46 47 (England and Wales); 08454 24 24 24 (Scotland)). Their experts may be able to find it for you.

If there is no reliable information to answer your question, ask NHS Direct whether anyone is currently preparing a systematic review of existing evidence, or whether there are any potentially relevant ongoing controlled trials.

If there is a relevant ongoing trial, consult www.controlled-trials.com or the specific trial website to see whether you can participate in it, and with whom you can discuss your options.

Agree to participate in a clinical trial only on condition (i) that the study protocol has been registered publicly on www.controlled-trials.com; (ii) that the protocol refers to the systematic reviews of existing evidence showing that the trial is justified; and (iii) that you receive a written assurance that the full study results will be published, and sent to all participants who indicate that they wish to receive them.

If no one seems to be taking an interest in your inadequately answered questions about the effects of treatments, submit them for consideration to the NHS Health Technology Assessment (HTA) Programme (www.ncchta.org), the National Institute for Health and Clinical Excellence (NICE) (www.nice.org.uk), and relevant medical research charities (www.amrc.org.uk).

Learn to recognise uncertainty; speak up; ask questions; seek honest answers.

Let your doctors know if you want to discuss evidence on the effects of treatments, and what uncertainties there are about them. You may find the information at www.ohri.ca/DecisionAid helpful.

Encourage wider education about the effects of biases and the play of chance, and lobby your MP and others about including this in the curriculum, beginning at primary school.

Be a healthy sceptic about unfounded claims and media reports of treatment 'breakthroughs'; ask pertinent questions; discuss with your friends.

Challenge treatments offered to you or your family on the basis of beliefs and dogmas, but unsubstantiated by reliable evidence.

Encourage and work with doctors, researchers, research funders, and others who are trying to promote research addressing inadequately answered questions about the effects of treatment which you regard as important.

REFERENCES

pages 1–14

1 Silverman WA. *Where's the evidence?* Oxford: Oxford University Press, 1998, p165.
2 Tallis R. *Enemies of hope: a critique of contemporary pessimism.* London: Macmillan, 1997.
3 Lock S. Medicine in the second half of the twentieth century. In: Loudon I, ed. *Western medicine: an illustrated history.* Oxford: Oxford University Press, 1997.
4 Chalmers I. Unbiased, relevant, and reliable assessments in healthcare. *British Medical Journal* 1988;317:1167–8. Citing Bunker JP, Frazier HS, Mosteller F. Improving health: measuring effects of medical care. *Milbank Quarterly,* 1994;72:2225–58.
5 Chalmers I. Evaluating the effects of care during pregnancy and childbirth. In: Chalmers I, Enkin M, Keirse MJNC, eds. *Effective care in pregnancy and childbirth.* Oxford: Oxford University Press, 1989:3–38.
6 Ulfelder H. The stilbestrol disorders in historical perspective. *Cancer* 1980;45: 3008–11.
7 Office of Technology Assessment. Identifying health technologies that work: searching for evidence. Washington, DC: US Government Printing Office, 1994.
8 Vandenbroucke JP. Thalidomide: an unanticipated adverse event. Available from: www.jameslindlibrary.org [accessed 5 December 2005].
9 Thomson D, Capstick T. How a risk management programme can ensure safety in thalidomide use. *Pharmaceutical Journal* 2004 Feb 14:194–5.
10 Melville A, Johnson C. *Cured to death: the effects of prescription drugs.* London: New English Library, 1983.
11 Anonymous. After practolol [Editorial]. *British Medical Journal* 1977; 17 Dec: 1561–2.
12 Chalmers I. Trying to do more good than harm in policy and practice: the role of rigorous, transparent, up-to-date evaluations. *Annals of the American Academy of Political and Social Science* 2003;589:22–40.
13 Furberg CD. Effect of antiarrhythmic drugs on mortality after myocardial infarction. *American Journal of Cardiology* 1983;52:32C–36C.
14 Chalmers I. In the dark. Drug companies should be forced to publish all the results of clinical trials. How else can we know the truth about their products. *New Scientist* 2004, 6 Mar, p19. Citing Moore T, *Deadly Medicine.* New York: Simon and Schuster, 1995.

15 Cowley AJ, Skene A, Stainer K, Hampton JR. The effect of lorcainide on arrhythmias and survival in patients with acute myocardial infarction: an example of publication bias. *International Journal of Cardiology* 1993;40:161–6.

16 Horn J, Limburg M. Calcium antagonists for acute ischemic stroke. *The Cochrane Database of Systematic Reviews* 2000, Issue 1. Art. No.: CD001928. Available from: www.thecochranelibrary.com [accessed 3 January 2006].

17 Horn J, de Haan RJ, Vermeulen PD, Luiten PGM, Limburg M. Nimodipine in animal model experiments of focal cerebral ischemia: a systematic review. *Stroke* 2001;32:2433–8.

18 Hemminki E, McPherson K. Impact of postmenopausal hormone therapy on cardiovascular events and cancer: pooled data from clinical trials. *British Medical Journal* 1997;315:149–53.

19 Anonymous. HRT: update on the risk of breast cancer and long-term safety. *Current Problems in Pharmacovigilance* 2003;29:1–3. Citing results of Women's Health Initiative randomised controlled trial (*Journal of the American Medical Association* 2003;289:3243–53) and Million Women Study (*Lancet* 2003;362: 419–27).

20 Williams HC. Evening primrose oil for atopic dermatitis: time to say goodnight [Editorial]. *British Medical Journal* 2003;327:1358–59.

21 Hoare C, Li Wan Po A, Williams H. Systematic review of treatment for atopic eczema. Health Technology Assessment Report 2000, volume 4, no. 37.

22 Takwale A, Tan E, Agarwal S, *et al*. Efficacy and tolerability of borage oil in adults and children with atopic eczema: randomised, double blind, placebo controlled, parallel group trial. *British Medical Journal* 2003;327:1385–87.

23 Wilks D, Sissons JGP. Infection. In: Tomlinson S, Heagerty AM, Weetman AP, eds. *Mechanisms of disease: an introduction to clinical science*. Cambridge: Cambridge University Press 1997, pp189–200.

24 Vandenbroucke JP, de Craen AJM. Alternative medicine: a 'mirror image' for scientific reasoning in conventional medicine. *Annals of Internal Medicine* 2001;135:507–13. Citing Ziegler EJ, Fisher CJ Jr, Sprung CL, *et al*. Treatment of gram-negative bacteremia and septic shock with HA-1A human monoclonal antibody against endotoxin. A randomized, double-blind, placebo-controlled trial. The HA-1A Sepsis Study Group. *New England Journal of Medicine* 1991;324:429–36 and citing Bone RC. Immunologic dissonance: a continuing evolution in our understanding of the systemic inflammatory response syndrome (SIRS) and the multiple organ dysfunction syndrome (MODS). *Annals of Internal Medicine* 1996;125:680–7.

25 Crile G. A plea against blind fear of cancer. *Life*, 1955, Oct 31, pp128–32.

26 Baum M, Houghton J. Contribution of randomised controlled trials to understanding and management of early breast cancer. *British Medical Journal* 1999;319:568–71.

27 Early Breast Cancer Trialists' Collaborative Group. Effects of adjuvant tamoxifen and of cytotoxic therapy on mortality in early breast cancer. An overview of 61 randomised trials among 28,896 women. *New England Journal of Medicine* 1988;319:1681–92.

28 Kolata G, Eichenwald K. Health business thrives on unproven treatment, leaving science behind. *New York Times* Special Report, 1999, Oct 2.

29 Farquhar C, Marjoribanks J, Basser R, *et al*. High dose chemotherapy and autologous bone marrow or stem cell transplantation versus conventional chemotherapy for women with early poor prognosis breast cancer. *The Cochrane Database of Systematic Reviews* 2005, Issue 3. Art. No.: CD003139. Available from: www.thecochranelibrary.com [accessed 3 January 2006].

30 Farquhar C, Marjoribanks J, Basser R, *et al*. High dose chemotherapy and autologous bone marrow or stem cell transplantation versus conventional chemotherapy for

women with metastatic breast cancer. *The Cochrane Database of Systematic Reviews* 2005, Issue 3. Art. No.: CD003142. Available from: www.thecochranelibrary.com [accessed 3 January 2006].

31 Thornton H. The screening debates: time for a broader approach? *European Journal of Cancer* 2003;39:1807–9.

32 Adapted from Wilson JMG, Jungner G. Principles and practice of screening for disease. Public health paper no 34. Geneva: World Health Organisation, 1968.

33 Gray JAM. *Evidence-based healthcare*. Edinburgh: Churchill Livingstone, 1997.

34 Morris JK. Screening for neuroblastoma in children. *Journal of Medical Screening* 2002;9:56.

35 Welch HG. *Should I be tested for cancer? Maybe not and here's why.* Berkeley and Los Angeles: University of California Press, 2004. p77.

36 Morris JK. Screening for neuroblastoma in children. *Journal of Medical Screening* 2002;9:56.

37 Hummel S, Paisley S, Morgan A, *et al.* Clinical and cost-effectiveness of new and emerging technologies for early localised prostate cancer: a systematic review. Health Technology Assessment Report 2003; volume 7, no. 33.

38 Law M. Screening without evidence of efficacy. *British Medical Journal* 2004;328:301–2.

39 Yamey G, Wilkes M. The PSA storm. *British Medical Journal* 2002;324:431.

40 Wallis C. Atypical cystic fibrosis – diagnostic and management dilemmas. *Journal of the Royal Society of Medicine* 2003;96(suppl 43):2–10.

41 David TJ. Newborn screening for cystic fibrosis. *Journal of the Royal Society of Medicine* 2004;97: 209–10.

42 Farrell MH, Farrell PM. Newborn screening for cystic fibrosis: ensuring more good than harm. *Journal of Pediatrics* 2003;143:707–12.

43 NICE. Guidance on the removal of wisdom teeth, 2000. Available from: www.nice.org.uk/page.aspx?o=526 [accessed 4 December 2005].

44 Allen C, Glasziou P, Del Mar C. Bed rest: a potentially harmful treatment needing more careful evaluation. *Lancet* 1999;354:1229–33.

45 Antman EM, Lau J, Kupelnick B, Mosteller F, Chalmers TC. A comparison of results of meta-analysis of randomized control trials and recommendations of clinical experts. *Journal of the American Medical Association* 1992;268:240–8.

46 Asher R. Talking sense (Lettsonian lecture, 16 Feb, 1959). *Transactions of the Medical Society of London*, vol LXXV, 1958–59. Reproduced in: Jones, FA, ed. *Richard Asher talking sense*. London: Pitman Medical, 1972.

47 Noseworthy JH, Ebers GC, Vandervoort MK, *et al.* The impact of blinding on the results of a randomized, placebo-controlled multiple sclerosis clinical trial. *Neurology* 1994;44:16–20.

48 Antiplatelet Trialists' Collaborative Group. Collaborative overview of randomised trials of antiplatelet therapy. *British Medical Journal* 1994;308:81–106.

49 Beral V, for the Million Women Study Collaborators. Breast cancer and hormone-replacement therapy in the Million Women Study. *Lancet* 2003;362:419–27.

50 Address by the Rt. Hon. Lord Rayleigh. In: Report of the fifty-fourth meeting of the British Association for the Advancement of Science; held at Montreal in August and September 1884, London: John Murray, pp3–23.

51 Reynolds LA, Tansey EM, eds. Prenatal corticosteroids for reducing morbidity and mortality after preterm birth. London: Wellcome Trust Centre for the History of Medicine, 2005.

52 Lindley RI. Personal communication, 2005.

53 Druker BJ, Talpaz M, Resta DJ, *et al.* Efficacy and safety of a specific inhibitor of the BCR-ABL tyrosine kinase in chronic myeloid leukemia. *New England Journal of Medicine* 2001;344:1031–7.

54 Loudon I. The use of historical controls and concurrent controls to assess the effects

of sulphonamides, 1936–1945. Available from: www.jameslindlibrary.org [accessed 3 January 2006].

55 Transurethral resection of the prostate for benign prostatic hyperplasia. In: Wennburg JE, McAndrew Cooper M, eds. The Dartmouth Atlas of Healthcare in the United States. Hanover, New Hampshire: Center for Evaluative Clinical Sciences, Dartmouth Medical School, 1996, p142. The 1996 edition and the updated 1999 edition are available from: www.dartmouthatlas.org/atlases/atlas_series.shtm [accessed 29 December 2005].

56 Burton MJ, Towler B, Glasziou P. Tonsillectomy versus non-surgical treatment for chronic/recurrent acute tonsillitis. *The Cochrane Database of Systematic Reviews* 1999, Issue 3. Art. No.: CD001802. Available from: www.thecochranelibrary.com [accessed 3 January 2006].

57 Ashcroft R. Giving medicine a fair trial. *British Medical Journal* 2000;320:1686.

58 Smithells RW. Iatrogenic hazards and their effects. *Postgraduate Medical Journal* 1975;15:39–52.

59 General Medical Council. Seeking patients' consent: the ethical considerations. November 1998. Available from: www.gmc-uk.org/guidance/library/consent.asp [accessed 6 December 2005].

60 Chalmers I, Lindley R. Double standards on informed consent to treatment. In: Doyal L, Tobias JS, eds. *Informed consent in medical research*. London: BMJ Books 2001, pp266–75.

61 Goodare H. Studies that do not have informed consent from participants should not be published. In: Doyal L, Tobias JS, eds. *Informed consent in medical research*. BMJ Books 2001, pp131–3.

62 Fallowfield L, Jenkins V, Farewell V, *et al*. Efficacy of a Cancer Research UK communicating skills training model for oncologists: a randomised controlled trial. *Lancet* 2002;359:650–6.

63 Tobias J, Souhami R. Fully informed consent can be needlessly cruel. *British Medical Journal* 1993;307:119–20.

64 Baum, M. The ethics of randomised controlled trials. *European Journal of Surgical Oncology* 1995;21:136–7.

65 Thornton H. Why do we need clinical trials? *BACUP News*; issue 30, autumn 1997, p7.

66 de Takats P, Harrison J. Clinical trials and stroke. *Lancet* 1999;353:150.

67 Chalmers I, Lindley R. Double standards on informed consent to treatment. In: Doyal L, Tobias JS, eds. *Informed consent in medical research*. London: BMJ Books 2001, pp266–75.

68 Ashcroft, R. Giving medicine a fair trial. *British Medical Journal* 2000;320:1686.

69 Savulescu J, Chalmers I, Blunt J. Are research ethics committees behaving unethically? Some suggestions for improving performance and accountability. *British Medical Journal* 1996;313:1390–3.

70 European Carotid Surgery Trialists' Collaborative Group. Randomised trial of endarterectomy for recently symptomatic carotid stenosis: final results of the MRC European Carotid Surgery Trial (ECST). *Lancet* 1998;351:1379–87.

71 Cina CS, Clase CM, Haynes RB. Carotid endarterectomy for symptomatic carotid stenosis. *The Cochrane Database of Systematic Reviews* 1999, Issue 3. Art. No.: CD001081. Available from: www.thecochranelibrary.com [accessed 3 January 2006].

72 The Magpie Trial Collaborative Group. Do women with pre-eclampsia, and their babies, benefit from magnesium sulphate? The Magpie Trial: a randomised, placebo-controlled trial. *Lancet* 2002;359:1877–90.

73 Duley L, Gülmezoglu AM, Henderson-Smart DJ. Magnesium sulphate and other anticonvulsants for women with pre-eclampsia. *The Cochrane Database of Systematic Reviews* 2003, Issue 2. Art. No.: CD000025. Available from: www.thecochranelibrary.com [accessed 3 January 2006].

74 Grimwade K, Swingler, G, Grimley Evans J. Cotrimoxazole prophylaxis for opportunistic infections in adults with HIV. *The Cochrane Database of Systematic Reviews* 2003, Issue 3. Art. No.: CD003108. Available from: www.thecochranelibrary.com [accessed 3 January 2006].

75 Chintu C, Bhat GJ, Walker AS, *et al*. Co-trimoxazole as prophylaxis against opportunistic infections in HIV-infected Zambian children (CHAP): a double blind randomised placebo-controlled trial. *Lancet* 2004;364:1865–71.

76 MRC News Release. Antibiotic drug almost halves AIDS-related death in children. London: MRC, November 19, 2004.

77 Soares K, McGrath J, Adams C. Evidence and tardive dyskinesia. *Lancet* 1996;347:1696–7.

78 Thornley B, Adams C. Content and quality of 2000 controlled trials in schizophrenia over 50 years. *British Medical Journal* 1998;317:1181–4.

79 Howell CJ, Chalmers I. A review of prospectively controlled comparisons of epidural with non-epidural forms of pain relief during labour. *International Journal of Obstetric Anesthesia* 1992;1:93–110.

80 Chan A-W, Hróbjartsson A, Haahr MT, Gøtzsche PC, Altman DG. Empirical evidence for selective reporting of outcomes in randomized trials: comparison of protocols to published articles. *Journal of the American Medical Association* 2004;291:2457–65.

81 Horn J, de Haan RJ, Vermeulen RD, Luiten PGM, Limburg M. Nimodipine in animal model experiments of focal cerebral ischemia: a systematic review. *Stroke* 2001;32:2433–8.

82 Lau J, Schmid CH, Chalmers TC. Cumulative meta-analysis of clinical trials builds evidence of exemplary clinical practice. *Journal of Clinical Epidemiology* 1995;48: 45–57.

83 Altman DG. The scandal of poor medical research. *British Medical Journal* 1994;308:283–4.

84 Tallon D, Chard J, Dieppe P. Relation between agendas of the research community and the research consumer. *Lancet* 2000;355:2037–40.

85 Cream J, Cayton H. New drugs for Alzheimer's disease – a consumer perspective. *CPD Bulletin Old Age Psychiatry* 2001;2:80–2.

86 Cohen CI, D'Onofrio A, Larkin L, Berkholder P, Fishman H. A comparison of consumer and provider preferences for research on homeless veterans. *Community Mental Health Journal* 1999;35:273–9.

87 Griffiths KM, Jorm AF, Christensen H, *et al*. Research priorities in mental health, Part 2: an evaluation of the current research effort against stakeholders' priorities. *Australian and New Zealand Journal of Psychiatry* 2002;36:327–39.

88 Chalmers I. Current controlled trials: an opportunity to help improve the quality of clinical research. *Current Controlled Trials in Cardiovascular Medicine* 2000;1:3–8. Available from : http://cvm.controlled-trials.com/content/1/1/3 [accessed 12 December 2005].

89 Safeguarding participants in controlled trials [Editorial]. *Lancet* 2000;355:1455–63.

90 Weatherall D. Academia and industry: increasingly uneasy bedfellows. *Lancet* 2000;355:1574.

91 Angell M. Is academic medicine for sale? *New England Journal of Medicine* 2000;342:1516–8.

92 Grant J, Green L, Mason B. From bench to bedside: Comroe and Dripps revisited. HERG Research Report No. 30. Uxbridge, Middlesex: Brunel University Health Economics Research Group, 2003.

93 Pound P, Ebrahim S, Sandercock P, *et al*. Reviewing Animal Trials Systematically (RATS) Group. Where is the evidence that animal research benefits humans? *British Medical Journal* 2004;328:514–7.

94 Jones S. Genetics in medicine: real promises, unreal expectations [Milbank report].

New York: Milbank Memorial Fund, 2000. Available from: www.milbank.org [accessed 12 December 2005].

95 Mackillop WJ, Palmer MJ, O'Sullivan B, *et al*. Clinical trials in cancer: the role of surrogate patients in defining what constitutes an ethically acceptable clinical experiment. *British Journal of Cancer* 1989;59:388–95.

96 Jobling R. Therapeutic research into psoriasis: patients' perspectives, priorities and interests. In: Rawlins M, Littlejohns P, ed. *Delivering quality in the NHS 2005*. Abingdon: Radcliffe Publishing Ltd, pp53–6.

97 Dixon-Woods M. Agarwak S, Jones J, *et al*. Synthesising qualitative and quantitative evidence: a review of possible methods. *Journal of Health Services Research and Policy* 2005;10:45–53.

98 Koops L, Lindley RI. Thrombolysis for acute ischaemic stroke: consumer involvement in design of new randomised controlled trial. *British Medical Journal* 2002;325:415–7.

99 Donovan J, Mills N, Smith M, *et al*. Quality improvement report: improving design and conduct of randomised trials by embedding them in qualitative research: ProtecT (prostate testing for cancer and treatment) study. *British Medical Journal* 2002;325:766–9.

100 Edwards A, Elwyn G, Atwell C, *et al*. Shared decision making and risk communication in general practice – a study incorporating systematic literature reviews, psychometric evaluation of outcome measures, and quantitative, qualitative and health economic analyses of a cluster randomised trial of professional skill development. Report to 'Health in Partnership' programme, UK Department of Health. Cardiff: Department of General Practice, University of Wales College of Medicine, 2002.

101 Longo M, Cohen D, Hood K, *et al*. Involving patients in primary care consultations: assessing preferences using Discrete Choice Experiments. *British Journal of General Practice* 2006;56:35–42.

102 Marsden J, Bradburn J. Patient and clinician collaboration in the design of a national randomised breast cancer trial. *Health Expectations* 2004;7:6–17.

103 Warlow C, Sandercock P, Dennis M, Wardlaw J. Research funding. *Lancet* 1999;353:1626.

104 Chalmers I, Rounding C, Lock K. Descriptive survey of non-commercial randomised trials in the United Kingdom, 1980–2002. *British Medical Journal* 2003;327:1017–9.

105 Relman AS. Publications and promotions for the clinical investigator. *Clinical Pharmacology and Therapeutics* 1979;25:673–6.

106 Warlow C. Building trial capacity (in a hostile environment). Paper presented at Clinical Excellence 2004, Birmingham, 30 November 2004.

107 Eclampsia Trial Collaborative Group. Which anticonvulsant for women with eclampsia? Evidence from the Collaborative Eclampsia Trial. *Lancet* 1995;345:1455–63.

108 Alderson P, Roberts I. Corticosteroids for acute traumatic brain injury. *The Cochrane Database of Systematic Reviews* 2005, Issue 1. Art. No.: CD000196. Available from: www.thecochranelibrary.com [accessed 3 January 2006].

109 Roberts I, Yates D, Sandercock P, *et al*; CRASH trial collaborators. Effect of intravenous corticosteroids on death within 14 days in 10 008 adults with clinically significant head injury (MRC CRASH trial): randomised placebo-controlled trial. *Lancet* 2004;364:1321–8.

110 House of Commons Health Committee. The influence of the pharmaceutical industry. Fourth Report of Session 2004–2005. London: Stationery Office, 2005. Available from: www.publications.parliament.uk/pa/cm200405/cmselect/cmhealth/42/42.pdf [accessed 1 January 2006].

111 MRC announces plans for strengthening UK clinical research. MRC Network, Summer 2005.

112 Department of Health. Best research for best health: a new national health research strategy. London: Stationery Office, 2006. Available from www.dh.gov.uk/research

113 Cochrane Injuries Group Albumin Reviewers. Human albumin administration in critically ill patients: systematic review of randomised controlled trials. *British Medical Journal* 1998;317:235–40.

114 Finfer S, Bellomo R, Bryce N, *et al* (SAFE Study Investigators). A comparison of albumin and saline for fluid resuscitation in the intensive care unit. *New England Journal of Medicine* 2004;350:2247–56.

115 Tallon D, Chard J, Dieppe P. Relation between agendas of the research community and the research consumer. *Lancet* 2000;355:2037–40.

116 Hanley B, Truesdale A, King A, *et al*. Involving consumers in designing, conducting, and interpreting randomised controlled trials: questionnaire survey. *British Medical Journal* 2001;322:519–23.

117 Oliver S, Clarke-Jones L, Rees R, *et al*. Involving consumers in research and development agenda setting for the NHS: developing an evidence-based approach. *Health Technology Assessment* 2004;8:no.15.

118 Koops L, Lindley RI. Thrombolysis for acute ischaemic stroke: consumer involvement in design of new randomised controlled trial. *British Medical Journal* 2002;325:415–7.

119 Thornton H, Edwards A, Elwyn G. Evolving the multiple roles of 'patients' in health-care research: reflections after involvement in a trial of shared decision-making. *Health Expectations* 2003;6:189–97.

120 Chalmers I. Minimising harm and maximising benefit during innovation in healthcare: controlled or uncontrolled experimentation? *Birth* 1986;13;155–64.

121 Kushner R. *Breast cancer: a personal history and an investigative report*. New York: Harcourt Brace Jovanovitch, 1975.

122 Lerner BH. The breast cancer wars: hope, fear, and the pursuit of a cure in twentieth-century America. New York: Oxford University Press, 2003.

123 Faulder C. Always a woman: a practical guide to living with breast surgery. (Published in association with the Breast Care and Mastectomy Association). London: Thorsons, 1992, pp28–9;73;164–6.

124 Breast Cancer Care. Some of the most memorable events and milestones in our history. Available from: http://80.175.42.169/content.php?page_id=1338 [accessed 8 December 2005].

125 Institute of Medical Ethics Working Party on the ethical implications of AIDS: AIDS, ethics, and clinical trials. *British Medical Journal* 1992;305:699–701.

126 Thornton H. The patient's role in research. [Paper given at The Lancet 'Challenge of Breast Cancer' Conference, Brugge, April 1994.] In: Health Committee Third Report. *Breast cancer services. Volume II. Minutes of evidence and appendices*. London: HMSO, July 1995, 112–4.

127 Concorde Coordinating Committee. Concorde: MRC/ANRS randomised double-blind controlled trial of immediate and deferred zidovudine in symptom-free HIV infection. *Lancet* 1994;343:871–81.

128 Royal Courts of Justice. In the High Court of Justice, Family Division. Neutral citation [2002] EWHC 2734 (Fam). Cases nos: FD02p01866 & FD02p01867. 11 December 2002.

129 Herceptin and early breast cancer: a moment for caution [Editorial]. *Lancet* 2005;366:1673.

130 Hanley B, Truesdale A, King A, *et al*. Involving consumers in designing, conducting and interpreting randomised controlled trials: questionnaire survey. *British Medical Journal* 2001, 322:519–23.

131 Rice GPA, Incorvaia B, Munari L, *et al*. Interferon in relapsing-remitting multiple sclerosis. *The Cochrane Database of Systematic Reviews* 2001, Issue 4. Art. No.: CD002002. Available from: www.thecochranelibrary.com [accessed 3 January 2006].

132 Herxheimer A. Relationships between the pharmaceutical industry and patients' organisations. *British Medical Journal* 2003;326:1208–10.

133 Consumers' Association. Who's injecting the cash? *Which?* 2003, April, pp24–5.

134 Thornton H, Edwards A, Elwyn G. Evolving the multiple roles of 'patients' in health-care research: reflections after involvement in a trial of shared decision-making. *Health Expectations* 2003;6;189–97.

135 Koops L, Lindley RI. Thrombolysis for acute ischaemic stroke: consumer involvement in design of new randomised controlled trial. *British Medical Journal* 2002;325:415–7.

136 Hamdy FC. The ProtecT Study (Prostate testing for cancer and Treatment), 2001. Available from: www.shef.ac.uk/dcss/medical/urology/research/topic2.html [accessed 8 December 2005].

137 Oliver S, Clarke-Jones L, Rees R, *et al.* Involving consumers in research and development agenda setting for the NHS: developing an evidence-based approach. *Health Technology Assessment* 2004;8:no.15.

138 Minot GR, Murphy WP. Treatment of pernicious anemia by a special diet. *Journal of the American Medical Association* 1926;87:470–6.

139 House of Commons Health Committee. The influence of the pharmaceutical industry. Fourth Report of Session 2004–05. London: Stationery Office, 2005. Available from: www.publications.parliament.uk/pa/cm200405/cmselect/cmhealth/42/42.pdf [accessed 1 January 2006].

ADDITIONAL RESOURCES

DO YOU WANT ADDITIONAL GENERAL INFORMATION ABOUT TESTING TREATMENTS?

Websites

The James Lind Library
www.jameslindlibrary.org

NHS Choices
www.nhs.uk (enter 'research' in search window)

UK Clinical Research Collaboration
www.ukcrc.org/publications/informationbooklets

DIPEx Foundation
www.healthtalkonline.org

US National Cancer Institute
cancertrials.nci.nih.gov/clinicaltrials/learning

Blogs

Margaret McCartney blogs.ft.com/healthblog

Ben Goldacre www.badscience.net

Books

Ben Goldacre (2009). Bad science. London: Harper Perennial

Bengt Furberg and Curt Furberg CD (2007). Evaluating clinical research: all that glitters is not gold. 2nd edition. New York: Springer.

Steven Woloshin, Lisa Schwartz and Gilbert Welch (2008). Know your chances: understanding health statistics. Berkeley: University of California Press.

Druin Burch (2009). Taking the medicine. London: Chatto and Windus.

Irwig L, Irwig J, Trevena L, Sweet M (2008). Smart Health Choices. London: Hammersmith Press.

DO YOU WANT INFORMATION ABOUT WHAT IS KNOWN ABOUT THE EFFECTS OF TREATMENTS?

NHS Evidence
www.evidence.nhs.uk

DO YOU WANT INFORMATION ABOUT WHAT ISN'T KNOWN ABOUT THE
EFFECTS OF TREATMENTS?

UK Database of Uncertainties about the Effects of Treatments (UK DUETs) www.library.nhs.uk/duets

DO YOU WANT INFORMATION ABOUT ONGOING RESEARCH ADDRESSING
UNCERTAINTIES ABOUT THE EFFECTS OF TREATMENTS?

WHO International Clinical Trials Registry Platform
www.who.int/ictrp/en

DO YOU WANT TO BECOME INVOLVED IN IMPROVING THE RELEVANCE AND
QUALITY OF RESEARCH ON THE EFFECTS OF TREATMENTS?

James Lind Alliance
www.lindalliance.org
Promotes working partnerships between patients and clinicians to identify and
prioritise important uncertainties about the effects of treatments.

NIHR Health Technology Assessment
www.ncchta.org/sundry/infosheets/consumers.rtf
Actively involves service-users in all stages of its work.

Cochrane Consumer Network
www.cochrane.org/consumers/homepage.htm
Promotes patient input to systematic reviews of treatments prepared by The
Cochrane Collaboration.

UK Clinical Research Network
www.ukcrn.org.uk

WOULD YOU LIKE TO RECEIVE TRAINING INTRODUCING YOU TO THE
ASSESSMENT OF RESEARCH?

Critical Appraisal Skills Programme
http://www.phru.nhs.uk/pages/PHD/CASP.htm
Organises workshops and other resources to help individuals to develop the
skills to find and make sense of research evidence.

United States Cochrane Center
Understanding Evidence-based Healthcare: A Foundation for Action.
http://apps1.jhsph.edu/cochrane/CUEwebcourse.htm
A web course designed to help individuals understand the fundamentals of
evidence-based healthcare concepts and skills.

TRANSLATIONS OF TESTING TREATMENTS

Testing Treatments has been translated into Arabic, Chinese, German, Italian,
and Spanish. For further information go to www.jameslindlibrary.org

INDEX

co-trimoxazole 63–4
colds 36, 98
commercial pressures 8, 18–19, 23, 32, 75
    eclampsia 76
    evening primrose oil 11, 43
    interferons 90
    me-too drugs 70–2
    steroids 77
comparisons 29–32
    avoiding bias 32–5
    interpretation 37–8
computed tomography (CT) 1
confidence intervals 38, 39
cot death 7, 8
Creutzfeld-Jakob disease (CJD) 54–5, 87–8
cystic fibrosis 24–5, 72
cytokines 11–12

D
deafness 6
dentistry 26
depression 6, 70
diabetes 30, 47
diethylstilboestrol (DES) 4, 30
diphtheria 1
DNA 71–2
doctors 3, 6, 12, 14, 16, 100
    bias 35, 57
    screening 19, 22–4
    uncertainty 45–6, 52–3, 56–7
Down syndrome 22
drugs 1, 4–6, 70
    licensing 6, 11, 38, 71
    me-too drugs 70–1
    testing 6–7, 7–8

E
eclampsia 63, 64, 76
eczema 9–10, 43
electronic journals 42
endotoxins 11–12
epidurals 66
erysipelas 49
ethics 56, 57, 59–61
evening primrose oil 9–11, 43
evidence 2, 3, 18, 23
    assessing 40–1
    ignoring 32
    reviewing 7–9, 31–2, 42–3, 99
    uncertainty 46
    eye damage 6

F
Food and Drug Administration 90

G
gamma linolenic acid (GLA) 9–11
General Medical Council 56
glatiramer 89

H
Health, Department of 11, 89
    Committee on Safety of Medicines 6
healthcare 2, 25, 50
heart attacks 1, 7, 9, 27, 34, 38
    arrhythmia 7–8, 31, 41
    aspirin 38, 40
heart disease 5–6
Herceptin (trastuzumab) 88
high blood pressure 1, 63
High Court 87–8
hip replacements 30, 47, 49
HIV (human immunodeficiency virus) 63–4, 85, 87
hormone replacement therapy (HRT) 9, 10, 33–4, 70
    breast cancer 40
House of Commons Select Committee on Health 77, 100
housing 2

I
ibuprofen 70
imaging techniques 1
imatinib 47–8
immune system 11–12
information 82, 85
    overload 69
    patients 58, 84
insulin 30, 47
interferons 88–90

J
James Lind Library *xi*, 29
joint replacements 2

K
key points 13, 27, 44, 61, 68, 78, 95

L
laboratory research 71, 75
leukaemia 1, 47–8
life expectancy 2, 25

ultrasound 1
uncertainty 29, 45–6, 53–5, 56–7, 74,
        98–9
    benign prostatic hyperplasia 49–50
    breast cancer 52
    prostate cancer 50, 51, 74
    tonsillectomy 50–1
UNICEF 64
universities 71, 75

V
vaginal cancer 4
Vietnam War 8

vitamin B12 47, 49, 96–8
vitamin C 3

W
water 2
wisdom teeth 26
World Health Organisation 20, 64, 76

Y
Yellow Card scheme 6

Z
zidovudine 86–7

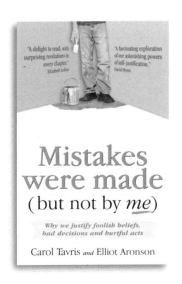

Mistakes were made (but not by me)
Carol Tavris & Elliot Aronson

2008 | paperback | 304 pages | ISBN 978-1-905177-21-9

Why do people dodge responsibility when things fall apart? Why the parade of public figures unable to own up when they make mistakes? Why the endless marital quarrels over who is right? Why can we see hypocrisy in others but not in ourselves? Are we all liars? Or do we really believe the stories we tell?

Renowned social psychologists Carol Tavris and Elliot Aronson take a compelling look into how the brain is wired for self-justification. When we make mistakes, we must calm the cognitive dissonance that jars our feelings of self-worth. And so we create fictions that absolve us of responsibility, restoring our belief that we are smart, moral, and right – a belief that often keeps us on a course that is dumb immoral, and wrong. Backed by years of research and delivered in lively, energetic prose, *Mistakes Were Made (But Not by Me)* offers a fascinating explanation of self-deception – how it works, the harm it can cause, and how we can overcome it.

"**Fascinating.**" Financial Times

"**Excellent.**" The Guardian

"**A brilliant new book.**" The Times

"**By turns entertaining, illuminating and – when you recognise yourself in the stories it tells – mortifying.**" The Wall Street Journal

read an extract at **www.pinterandmartin.com/reading-room**

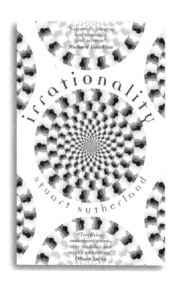

Irrationality
Stuart Sutherland

2007 | paperback | 256 pages | ISBN 978-1-905177-07-3

Why do doctors, army generals, high-ranking government officials, and other people in positions of power make bad decisions that cause harm to others? On the other hand, why do people insist on sitting through an awful play or film just because the tickets were expensive?

Irrational beliefs and behaviour are virtually universal. It is not only gamblers and parapsychologists that fall into simple statistical traps to do with sample sizes or simple assumptions, but experts of all types, selection committees, and everyday people. *Irrationality* is an iconoclastic volume that draws on a mass of intriguing research to examine why we are irrational, the different types of irrationality, the damage it does us, and the possible cures. It also argues that we could significantly reduce irrationality and its effects – but only if we first recognize just how irrational we really are.

"Superb! The thinking man's self help book; it left me infinitely wiser, but I know it won't change my behaviour one tiny bit."
BEN GOLDACRE, author of *Bad Science*

"Terrifying, sometimes comic, very readable and totally enthralling." OLIVER SACKS

"Extremely gripping and unusually well written." RICHARD DAWKINS

read an extract at **www.pinterandmartin.com/reading-room**

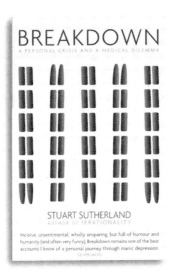

Breakdown
Stuart Sutherland

2010 | paperback | 356 pages | ISBN 978-1-905177-20-2

This acclaimed account by Stuart Sutherland, the best-selling author of *Irrationality*, of his own manic depression remains unique in its honesty and perception. As an eminent psychologist who suffered a severe mental breakdown, Sutherland provides us with an original and insightful description of his illness, its often bizarre consequences, and an analysis of the origins of mental illness.

Essential reading for students and anyone affected by or interested in mental illness, Sutherland describes and critically assesses the various forms of therapy and drug treatments available to sufferers of manic depression.

"Incisive, unsentimental, whole unsparing, but full of humour and humanity (and often very funny), Breakdown remains one of the best accounts I know of a personal journey through manic depression. I think it will take its place among the modern classics of this literature." OLIVER SACKS

"This is a book unlike any other that I have read. It combines a searingly honest and terrifyingly detailed account of a mental breakdown with a professional's description of the reality of mental illness as it is treated in our society. It is unforgettable. That is what a breakdown is really like." KINGLSEY AMIS

read an extract at **www.pinterandmartin.com/reading-room**

also from **Pinter & Martin**

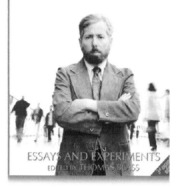

The Individual in a Social World
Stanley Milgram
paperback | ISBN 978-1-905177-12-7

When Prophecy Fails
Festinger, Riecken, Schachter
paperback | ISBN 978-1-905177-19-6

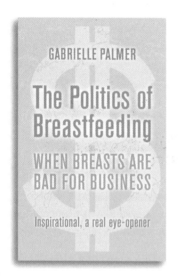

The Politics of Breastfeeding
Gabrielle Palmer
paperback | ISBN 978-1-905177-16-5

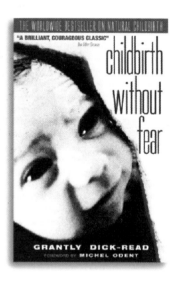

Childbirth without Fear
Grantly Dick-Read
paperback | ISBN 978-0-9530964-6-6

visit **www.pinterandmartin.com**
for further information, extracts and special offers